Doctor's Kitchen
3-2-1

3 PORTIONS OF FRUIT AND VEG

SERVING 2 PEOPLE

IN 1 PAN

DR RUPY AUJLA

Thorsons

Contents

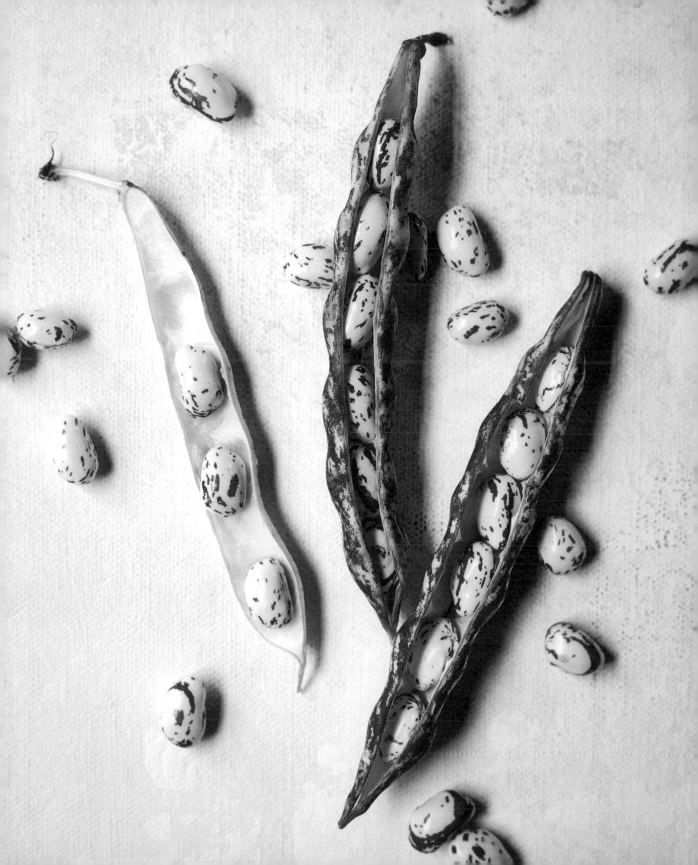

Introduction

Welcome to the wonderful world of 3-2-1! My name is Dr Rupy Aujla, NHS medical doctor, home cook and food as medicine advocate.

What is 3-2-1?

It's a brand new way of cooking delicious food that will completely change your life. Every recipe is formulated to contain **3 portions** of fruit and vegetables per person, each meal serves **2 people** and only requires **1 cooking pan** (like a roasting tray, saucepan or casserole dish) … that's it!

3-2-1 is my formula to produce incredible meals that taste spectacular, ensure health benefits to optimise and maintain your wellbeing, and streamline the cooking process so you can achieve healthy meals every single day. I know it sounds too good to be true, but I guarantee that this book will revolutionise the way you cook at home forever. It will become your go-to book for quick, no-fuss, wonderful food, which offers multiple benefits to your health.

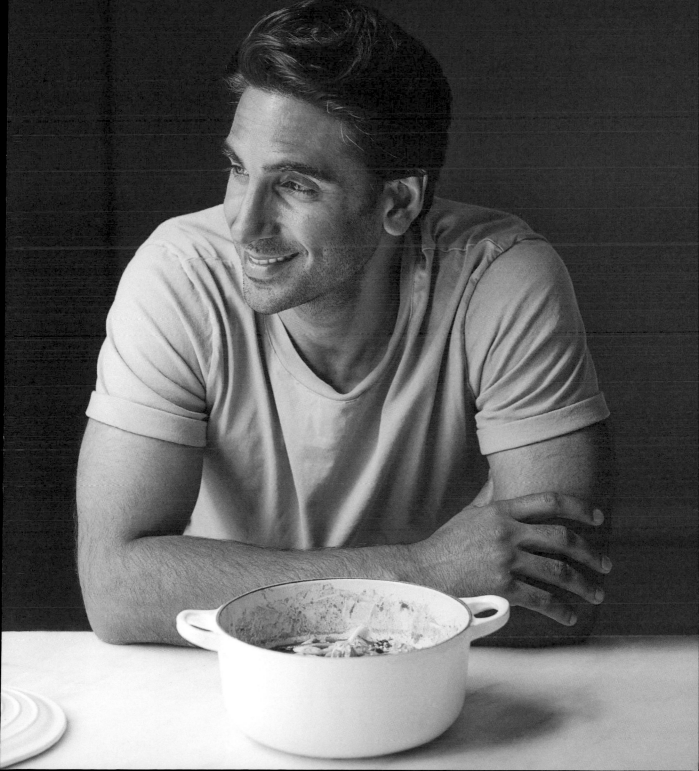

Why 3-2-1?

Over the last 5 years I've read hundreds of academic studies that examine what makes food beneficial to our wellbeing: which diets have been proven to have the biggest impact on health, which ingredients we need to include in our diets, the cooking processes that maintain their nutritional quality, and even the eating habits of the longest living and healthiest people on the planet.

From the research it is clear that the best thing we can do for our health is to focus on simply increasing the quantity and variety of fruits, nuts, seeds and vegetables in our diet.

It doesn't have to be about sticking to a particular dietary regimen, eating specific 'superfood' ingredients, obsessing about the proportion of macronutrients or calorie counting. And neither does it have to be solely about removing junk food, excess sugar and poor-quality fats from our plates (though we obviously still need to do this!); we need to focus on what our diets lack. A daily 'dose' of fresh wholesome plants, quality fats, wholegrains and plenty of fibre is what matters most, and 3-2-1 is your easy-to-follow daily prescription for good health.

FOOD AS MEDICINE

The benefits of dietary change are far ranging and I have discussed many topics like this in my last book, *Eat to Beat Illness*, as well as on my podcast, 'The Doctor's Kitchen'. In both, I cover in depth the incredible research that demonstrates the wide-ranging impact of nutritional medicine. Many leading institutes, including the World Health Organisation, recognise that eating a wholesome diet with plenty of fruit, vegetables, wholegrains, nuts and seeds, while limiting sugar, refined carbohydrates, poor-quality fats and animal products, lowers the

Our food can change our brain, alter our mood, support our immune function and reduce inflammation.

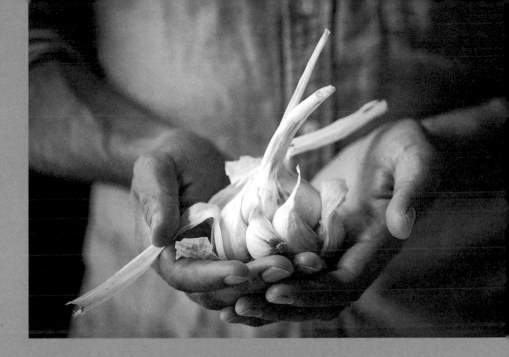

risk of a plethora of diseases including kidney failure, blindness caused by degenerative eye disease, cancer, depression, autoimmune conditions, obesity, heart disease and more.

Eating well is not just about removing foods that potentially cause disease, it's about consuming foods that amplify our defences against getting ill in the first place. There is a wealth of information on your plate that communicates with your inner ecosystem in the most powerful way imaginable. And we all have the opportunity to influence our health positively with the simple action of eating well. Frankly, we do not eat enough of the health-promoting ingredients that line our supermarket and grocery shelves in this country and beyond, and with this book I want to radically change that.

EATING WELL EVERY DAY

While this sounds painfully simple, the reality is that people still find it hard to eat well every day, myself included, which is why this book is geared towards helping you stick to eating well and developing a way of eating that you can enjoy and maintain in the long term. In a word, it's about consistency. We are constantly bombarded with fast-food outlets, convenience options and quick-fix diets, so it's no wonder many of us struggle to maintain a healthy diet and lifestyle. This is where I believe 3-2-1 can have a massive impact on your daily cooking habits and, ultimately, your health. Not only will this book help cultivate your inner chef, it will also help you to create plates that play a key part in the long-term health of you and your family that are sustainable.

How 3-2-1 works

What I've gained from the incredible opportunity of writing books, seeing thousands of patients in clinic and speaking to people at conferences, is the ability to listen and take action on feedback. And, let me assure you, I've listened to the feedback.

1 Each recipe provides more than adequate portions of 3 incredible and accessible foods. You'll begin to appreciate the wonderful benefits of the 'normal' fruits, vegetables, legumes, nuts and seeds that line our grocery and supermarket shelves. These are key to good health.

2 Every recipe serves 2 people, and to serve 4 you just double the ingredients.

3 Each meal requires only 1 pan. This helps save your mental energy, reduces the washing up and drastically lowers the hurdle of having to cook for yourself after a long day.

4 The recipes are streamlined to use as little equipment as possible. In fact, I've made sure that the majority of the recipes only require a good chef's knife and chopping board, and a frying pan, baking tray or decent casserole dish.

5 The recipes are very flexible: there are lots of substitution ideas, 'cheat' versions with fewer ingredients, and the recipes can be scaled up for family cook-ups, too – just double the ingredients to create a 3-2-1 meal for 4 people or even for batch cooking them at the start of the week.

6 By scanning the QR code on the recipe pages, you can transform the ingredient lists into a digital shopping list on your phone, making the recipes super easy to shop for.

It's more straightforward, achievable and enjoyable than you could ever imagine, and I hope to encourage you to at least consider a daily Doctor's Kitchen dinner.

I have also created the '3-2-1 week Kickstarter' (see page 52). In only 15 minutes of prep a day, you'll have breakfast, lunch and dinner sorted and it will kickstart your healthy-eating journey over one week. It's been a game changer for many of my colleagues, patients and friends, and I know it will help you too.

Keep it simple

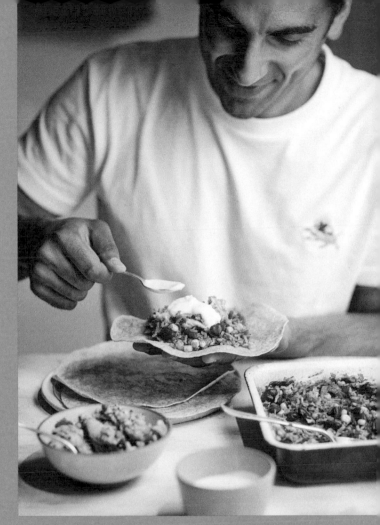

In an era of complexity and multiple 'authorities' to listen to, burgeoning nutritional science and controversy over which dietary dogma to follow, I'm keeping my message intentionally simple. I want you to understand the benefits of food and make changes today. I don't want to baffle you with complex terminology and over-promise when it comes to the benefits of dietary change. Diversifying your food is one of the easiest ways to improve health, and dotted throughout the book are sections on simple ingredients and their benefits, to inspire you about the beauty of whole foods and the medicinal impact of eating well: you'll learn why they're so healthful and about the research that underpins my firm belief in the power of food to prevent – and in some cases treat – ill health. It is my aim to help you effortlessly transform your cooking to support your wellbeing.

Simplifying life in the kitchen

I've tackled the main reasons why people choose not to cook at home and instead rely on the ever-increasing choices of convenience food:

Lack of mental energy

Waning motivation

Time and effort needed to create a meal

The dreaded washing up

As a busy doctor in the NHS who still works in emergency medicine doing shift work, I relate to the gruelling stresses and strains of maintaining healthy habits all too well. This is exactly why I've carefully curated each recipe and streamlined the cooking process to only involve one piece of cookware at a time, reduce preparation time and maximise flavour and function, while minimising faff.

Using just one pan creates a hassle-free method of cooking for when you struggle to find the motivation to prepare a meal for yourself after a hectic day. Nobody wants to be toasting nuts in one pan and juggling two saucepans on the hob, remembering to season and garnish each one after a stressful day. It's no wonder we crave the ease of a delivery!

3-2-1 is a new way of cooking that rises to the challenge of modern life without sacrificing the beauty of cooking, the process of creating incredibly satisfying meals and the nourishment of flavourful food. 3-2-1 recipes are designed to tick all the boxes.

- ☑ Speed
- ☑ Simplicity
- ☑ Indulgence
- ☑ Health benefits

By paring down life in the kitchen, I aim to give you back the most precious commodity of all: time. Time so you can look after both your physical and mental health and consider all the other lifestyle changes that can improve your wellbeing. This book will give you back time lost to the cooking process during the week, without compromising the health benefits of food or the enjoyment of it. 3-2-1 is now my mantra and I hope it resonates with you and guides you to effortlessly take care of your health.

Fast recipes versus smart recipes

When I ask patients and colleagues what they want from a healthy cookbook or meal plan, the most common answer is, 'I want it to be quick. 10 minutes or less' or even, 'I want it to be faster than my takeaway!' I could easily create the quickest recipe book of all time, but if the dishes involved multiple kitchen gadgets, chopping endless ingredients and finishing everything off in a couple of pans, your kitchen will be a mess, and you'd wear yourself out trying to focus on multiple things at once, which can lead to error and a stressful cooking experience! The process of cooking should be relaxing, especially at the end of a busy day, and what really works is *simplicity*: a cooking method that is frictionless, completely streamlined to the point where you do not need to overthink it. A method that delivers

peace of mind, fantastically flavoured and indulgent meals with the least effort. This is my most practical, easy-to-use book to date, and I know you and your family are going to love every single recipe.

We might not be professional chefs, culinary geniuses or nutrition experts, but many of us still want incredible-tasting and gorgeous-looking food. We want exquisitely balanced and nutritious dishes, and to be able to look after our bodies and beat illness by optimising our food choices. If these are the things you want, then this book is for you.

I'm so excited for you to join me in the kitchen, share this formula for good health and start cooking the 3-2-1 way! But before we launch into the cooking, I want to take you on a journey to convince you why we need to eat more, and the science of food as medicine that explains why a practising frontline medical doctor likes to write cookbooks.

By paring down life in the kitchen, I aim to give you back the most precious commodity of all: time.

Why we need to eat MORE

In an era where the phenomena of overindulgence on nutrient poor, energy-dense food is largely held accountable for the obesity epidemic sweeping through cities and towns across the globe, you may find the title of this chapter confusing. However, while it is true that high sugar, high fat, processed food litters our supermarket shelves and most public dining spaces, what is also just as prevalent is a distinct under-consumption of ingredients known to protect and promote our health. Fruit and vegetable consumption is drastically low, with an average daily intake of around 3 portions per person in the UK. But what is more revealing is that while the average intake is just over 3 portions a day, rates of consumption range between 5 and zero! Some of us are not having a single one of these ingredients that are critical to health and known to beat illness, and it breaks my heart. This chapter zooms in on why we need to eat more of these types of foods, where the evidence for such a simple message lies and how better research will yield more effective nutrition campaigns.

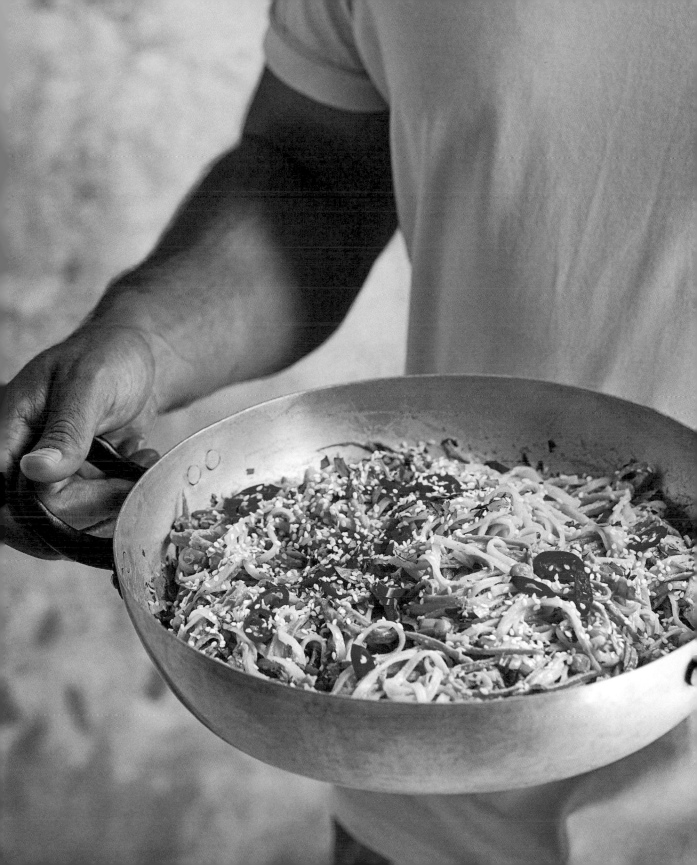

WHY '5-A-DAY' CAN BE PROBLEMATIC

The 5-a-day mantra is ingrained in our minds so effectively. Ask anyone how many fruit and vegetables they should be eating a day and without hesitation the answer will pop to the front of their mind: 5! Originally developed in the 1980s by Professor Ken Kizer and colleagues at California's State Department of Public Health Services, the campaign was enthusiastically welcomed by producers of fruit and vegetables in a bid to improve public health and the sales of their produce. Across different national healthcare systems, as well as the World Health Organisation (WHO), the same message was gradually adopted in response to a clear link between higher consumption of fruit and vegetables and a resulting lower risk of non-communicable diseases, including heart disease and cancer. Contributing evidence led to 400g being the general internationally agreed daily target for fruit and vegetable consumption, and the UK officially adopted the '5 a day' slogan (five 80g portions) in 2003.

While this slogan has been successful at informing the public on the minimum amount of fruit and vegetables to eat, our consumption is still very low. And despite the many aspirational, higher targets promoted by other countries, such as Japan's 13 and Australia's 7, the average consumption in those countries is very similar to ours, and well under 5. This is why I believe we need a new approach that focuses on behaviour change and strategies to ease the stress and time constraints of cooking with the goal of introducing more fruit and vegetables into our diet, rather than just reminding people to eat more portions. We need to focus on the nudges and behaviour changes that actually result in a significant increase in consumption of diverse plants. This is how 3-2-1 will help you, and millions of people, achieve this seemingly easy yet difficult-to-achieve habit.

The amount of fruit and veg you consume is the most critical component of good health.

WHY FRUIT AND VEG?

Hundreds of studies in nutritional science literature across multiple organisations around the world all point to the same association: the more fruits, vegetables, nuts and seeds in your diet, the lower the risk of disease across many areas including cancer, heart disease, diabetes, eye disease, mental health and more. Focusing your meals on plants and eating a greater variety of them is the mantra I've been reciting throughout all of my books – a 'plant-focused' approach of eating is the way to go, and 3-2-1 will show you how.

It may seem trivial and simplistic to focus on fruit and vegetable consumption alone, when there appear to be so many other variables that impact our health status. Some of those that are heavily advertised to us include calorie control, changing the proportions of macronutrients we consume (such as lowering carbs) or even alternate-day fasting. And while I appreciate the need to ensure we don't overconsume energy dense, nutrient poor food or eat a large proportion of high-sugar and refined carbohydrates, there is simply no other strategy at improving health and longevity that's more convincing than focusing on consuming more plants.

WHY NUTS AND SEEDS?

The value of increasing whole foods in your diet is not limited to fruit and vegetables alone, and that's why in this book I'm including the often overlooked, nutrient-dense nuts and seeds category as contributions to one of the '3' portions per recipe. Whether it's a handful of walnuts or a sprinkle of pumpkin seeds, these powerhouses of nutrition contain varied micronutrients including magnesium, vitamin E and beneficial plant chemicals that we need to eat more of.

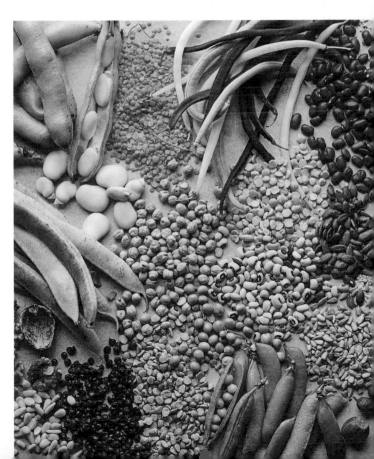

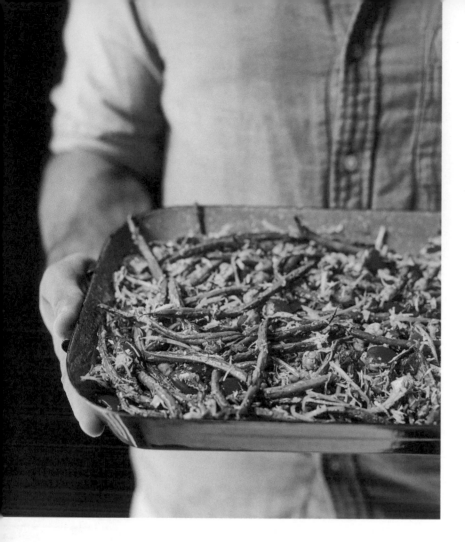

We now need
to make food
a priority in
medicine.

However, during an era in nutrition where all fats were considered to be 'bad', we have traditionally overlooked these types of foods because of their high fat content. The encouragement to eat these types of foods is lacklustre even today, because nutrition science is still bound to the paradigm of energy balance for weight control, and as nuts and seeds are high in fat, they are therefore high-calorie. There are fundamental flaws in this energy balance model that need to be addressed, but as was the case with fat versus sugar, it takes a while to change such ingrained, deeply held beliefs.

When analysing the research for nuts and seeds in the diet, it is clear that consuming them is associated with a reduction in the risk of chronic disease, and paradoxically is linked with better weight control – despite the high calorie content. More nuts and seeds in the diet is related to reduced cardiovascular disease and diabetes, and there is some research that demonstrates beneficial effects on cancer and high blood pressure. When it comes to these types of fats derived from whole ingredients, I truly believe we need to eat more of them. This is why nuts and seeds are on the menu and why they contribute a portion in the 3-2-1 recipes.

A BIT TOO EASY?

I understand that this sounds far too easy, but the data does not lie. Think of all the historical public health measures that have yielded the biggest impact on health and wellbeing: sanitation systems, clean drinking water and tobacco legislation are just a few examples of measures once thought to be drastic but now regarded as common sense and responsible for saving millions of lives. They were equally simplistic and hugely effective. Non-communicable diseases such as heart disease, obesity and stroke are now the biggest threat to health and cause most deaths in industrialised nations. Everybody appears to intrinsically know they should be eating more fruit and vegetables, and armed with the knowledge that fruit, vegetable, nut and seed consumption is key to reducing the risk of non-communicable diseases, we now need to make food a priority in medicine. We have an incredible opportunity to exponentially improve the health of our communities by encouraging positive food choices on a daily basis. Rather than having to wait for huge government campaigns and a shift in the mindset of medical practitioners, or even more evidence to add to the thousands of studies on this topic, this is a prescription you can fill in yourself, one delicious plate at a time.

THE NEED FOR BETTER NUTRITIONAL RESEARCH

The bias of modern medicine towards the use of pharmaceuticals is not because of a huge corporate conspiracy aimed at maximising profits. It is simply because it is far easier to perform research comparing one drug with another in a repeatable and methodical way that upholds the highest standards of scientific rigour. Comparing different diets is a completely different ball game and it's immensely tricky.

If you take the example of a seemingly simple study that tries to compare a 'low carbohydrate diet' to a 'high carbohydrate diet', you soon realise that many variations of each diet exist. How much sugar is there in each diet? What type of carbohydrate are they eating? Are there animal foods, and if so what type? How about the fat content? Is there more unsaturated versus saturated fat in each one? What time do the participants in the study eat? How many types of polyphenols are in each

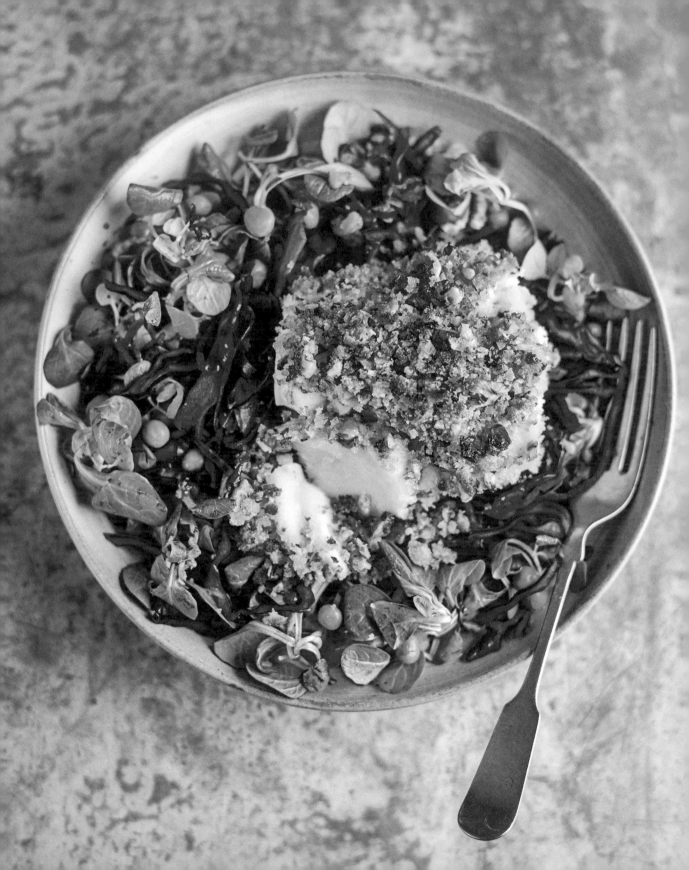

More vegetables in your diet results in better health outcomes.

meal? The list is endless, and that's before considering whether people can actually stick to the diet on a day-to-day basis for the duration of the study!

In addition, many nutrition studies are plagued by inconsistent methodology, lack of quality control, interpretation bias from the researchers themselves (who, for example, may be of a vegan or paleo persuasion), and that's before we consider how complex food is itself. A drug will typically affect a singular biological pathway, which makes a pharmaceutical product far simpler and easier to study, whereas food impacts multiple pathways simultaneously, including hormones, cellular metabolism, gut microbiota populations, inflammation and many others. This makes it incredibly hard to explain the mechanism of action of a diet and conclusively prove the benefits or negative impact of food to our physiology.

Furthermore, our current model of scientific research fails to appreciate 'behaviour change', which is indelibly tied to diet. There is no point

suggesting a diet that is expensive, restrictive or difficult to maintain in the long term despite its potential benefits, if people find it impossible to sustain. Consistency is key and the ease of complying with a diet, or any way of eating, needs to be considered before a recommendation is made to anyone.

Another aspect of diet that is difficult to capture in short-term research is how food choices can moderate risk or management of a disease over a long time period. Most high-quality nutrition studies occur over short periods of time, as they are limited by the huge cost of this type of research, and are simply not long enough to demonstrate meaningful results. But, if we are serious about using nutrition in medicine, we need to make considerable investments into long term, controlled studies rather than adding to the pool of lower quality research that dominates nutritional science.

Despite the pitfalls and complexity of nutrition research, there are plenty of legitimate and rigorous population studies and laboratory-based research, which – together with a new interest in ageing medicine, a good dose of common sense and my frontline clinical experience – strengthen my conviction in this plain and simple message: more vegetables in your diet results in better health outcomes. This is the underlying foundation that all dietary changes should be based on and why this book has been formulated to make that shift easier for you than ever.

MORE IS MORE

When we examine the research looking at fruit and vegetables and health outcomes the trend is fairly clear. There is a 'dose response' to eating vegetables, which is simply to say, the more the better. With each incremental increase in consumption, greater health protection is achieved. Researchers have found that the ideal amount of fruit and vegetable consumption is greater than 800g per day – that's equivalent to 10 portions. While that sounds wholly unachievable, it's actually equivalent to having three *Doctor's Kitchen 3-2-1* meals a day (where each meal consists of 3 portions of fruit and vegetables per person) plus a piece of fruit. The '3-2-1 week kickstarter' on page 52 will show you how to achieve this with just 15 minutes of prep a day, and hopefully this will encourage a new habitual way of cooking that will stick. The reality is, even if you can't achieve over 800g of fruit and vegetables a day, anything above 5 portions is fantastic.

Most of the recommendations for increasing fruit and vegetable consumption are based on epidemiological studies that observe associations between diet and health over time. This is one of the weaker methods of research and it cannot give us enough information to fully understand the impact of food on health. However, combining what we know of the link between food and health outcomes with studies looking at the potential mechanisms of how food impacts our physiology, there is a pretty clear case for it deserving more attention. I cover these studies in later chapters, but considering the limitations of nutritional science we need to be open minded and pragmatic about considering all the evidence looking at how food can be so impactful on health.

IT'S OUR RESPONSIBILITY

While the intention of the '5-a-day' message was to deliver a practical guide for consumers to make better health choices, and provide some clarity for producers on how to improve the nutrient density of their products, around the world there are some pretty loose definitions of what constitutes a portion. Pizza, tinned spaghetti and fruit juices have all been labelled as

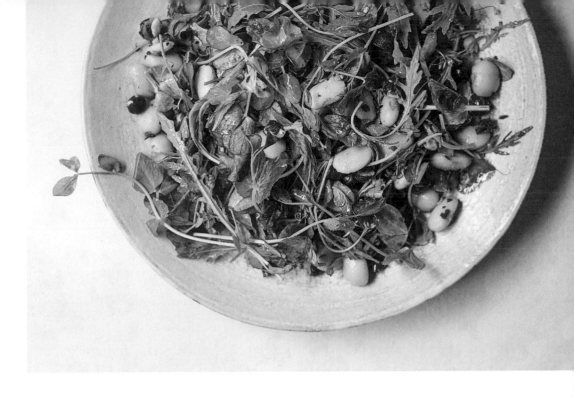

containing 'one of your 5 a day', and while technically it may be true, we have to consider a few things – such as how much processing a food has undergone or the addition of sugar, salt and other additives – in order to determine whether these are the types of foods you would want to consume regularly.

While I believe that working with the food industry is essential if we are going to make positive changes to our food landscape, it's clear that we cannot rely on industry alone to make these choices on our behalf and educate us appropriately. We have to be responsible for our own health. Everything in this book is geared towards getting proper fresh and wholesome ingredients into your diet and putting you in control of your health. There are no loose claims of portion sizes in this book, hence why the weights of ingredients are included, as well as described in amounts you would find in the supermarket (such as 2 small leeks or a bulb of fennel). I've done all the math to ensure that each meal contains a minimum of 3 portions of fruit, vegetables, nuts or seeds per serving, and every effort has been made to ensure the recipes stick to this promise throughout. The only way to be sure you're getting the nutrients you need to sustain your wellbeing is to put yourself in charge and cook from scratch (see page 50). That might sound like a daunting task, but 3-2-1 will show you how easy it can be.

Can you add just one more?

Small but consistent nutritious additions to your diet can spark huge changes to your overall way of eating that has the potential to improve multiple aspects of your health.

I want the sections dedicated to colourful ingredients dotted throughout this book to inspire you to add colour to every element of your meal, regardless of whether you are cooking a recipe from this book or enjoying another dish. These ingredients are key to good health and are full of complex compounds that have been demonstrated to impact our physiology in a powerful way. Eating more of them, and a variety of them, is what we need to focus on.

Perhaps you've ordered takeaway or you're in a restaurant and you want to increase the nutrient density of your meal to ensure a complete array of nutrients from different sides and pairings? Just add one more portion of fruit, vegetable, nut or seed to your plate at every mealtime and you will massively shift your dietary pattern towards a healthier one. That could mean ordering a side of plain wilted spinach in olive oil at a restaurant, or cooking a large batch of

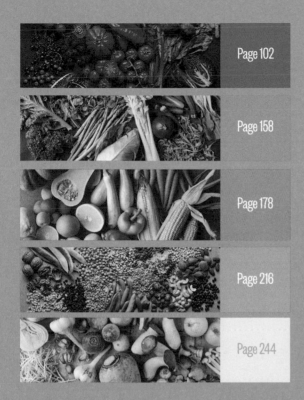

simply roasted asparagus spears and peppers as a delicious side to a pizza or another takeout. The 3-2-1 recipes are formulated so that you don't have to add extra vegetables to your meals, but for everything else, this is an easy guiding principle that works.

I know it seems basic, but with each incremental increase in portions of health-promoting whole foods, research tells us that we can hugely improve and protect our health. So just think to yourself at every mealtime, 'Can I add just one more?' The collective impact of these small actions could potentially lead to considerable health gains.

What portions look like

A bit of simple maths: every 3-2-1 recipe contains a minimum of 3 portions of different types of fruit, vegetables, nuts or seeds per person. As each recipe serves 2 people, there are – in total – 6 portions in each meal.

When you're out shopping for these ingredients I want to make it easier for you to recognise how vastly different 2 portions of fruit and vegetables appear.

The image on the next page is a selection of beans, nuts, seeds, fruits and vegetables in 2-portion sizes (i.e. the amounts commonly used in the recipes) to give you a better idea of how to 'eye' what portions look like when buying fresh produce in the shops.

A portion of fruit, vegetables and cooked legumes (such as black beans) is 80g, so 2 portions is 160g.

A portion of nuts, seeds and dried fruit is 30g, so 2 portions is 60g.

As you will see on the next page, 2 portions of watercress is vastly different to tomatoes or peaches in terms of size! And don't worry, the recipes are quite flexible, so feel free to use slightly more of each ingredient if it helps to minimise food waste.

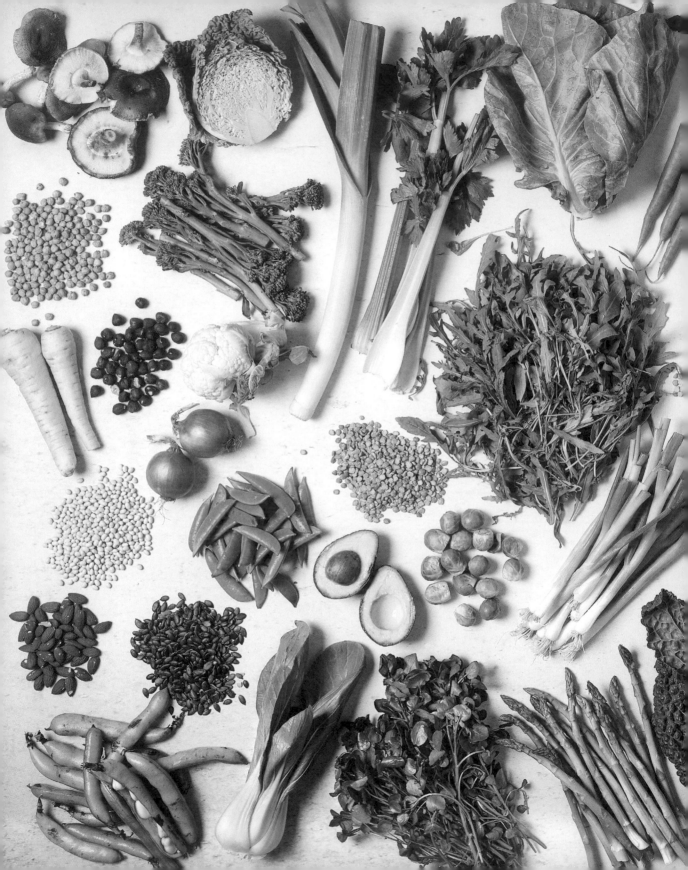

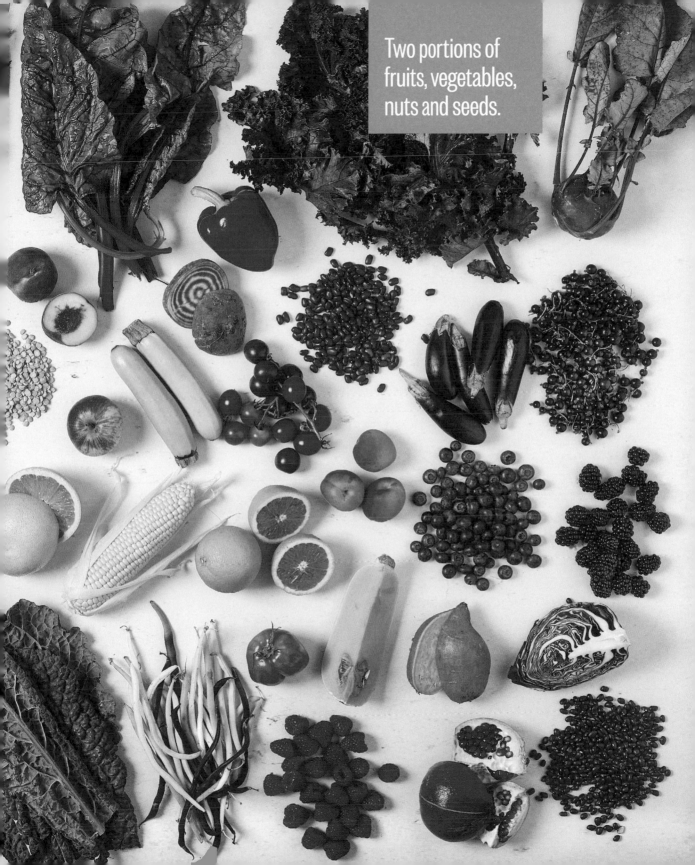

Two portions of fruits, vegetables, nuts and seeds.

Eat your medicine

My role as founder of The Doctor's Kitchen is to inspire you to eat well every day and remind you of the incredible physiological attributes gained by eating a wholesome diet. 'Food as medicine' promotes a perspective on the value of food beyond just whether something is a carbohydrate or is full of vitamins. As I said in my first book, food isn't a pill or a replacement for the pharmaceuticals and interventions I prescribe to patients daily, but it is an incredibly important tool in our clinical toolbox for the prevention of disease and promotion of wellbeing. To belittle medicine as just the prescription of pills and performance of surgery does not encompass the complexity and breadth of its practice.

Health professionals have a crucial role in nurturing a culture that recognises the power of food, and this is how we reverse the tidal wave of lifestyle-related disease that threatens to wipe out healthcare resources unless we address the root cause of illness. 'Food as medicine' is not a cute or quirky concept, but rather something I hope will become a clear and recognisable mainstream idea in the pursuit of a proactive, healthier population, a central idea that encourages health professionals to upskill and to be able to talk confidently about nutrition in all clinical settings (whether that be a hospital, psychiatric clinic or the community general practice), and a concept that encourages people to look after their health using food, knowing how impactful the ingredients we put on our plates are.

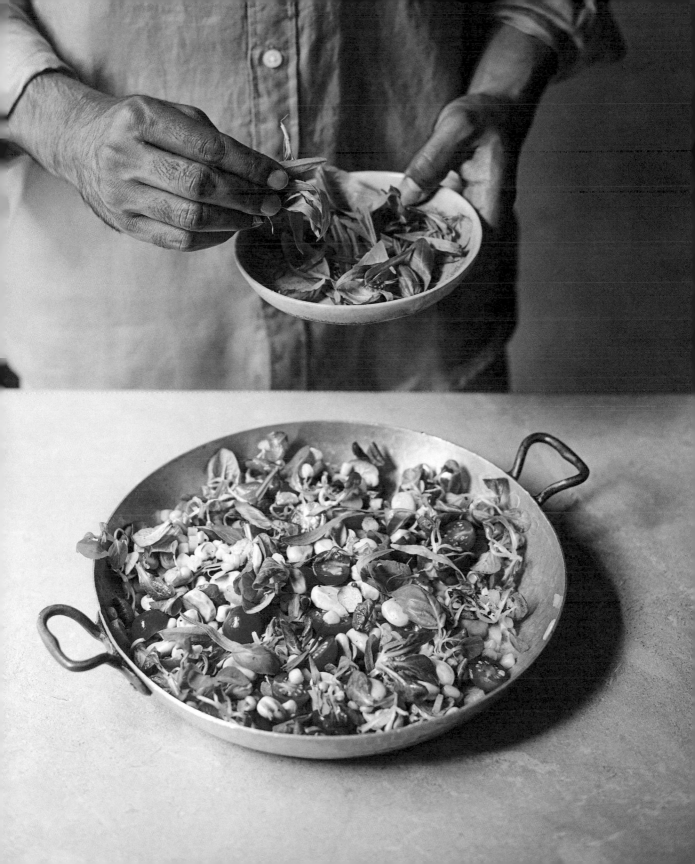

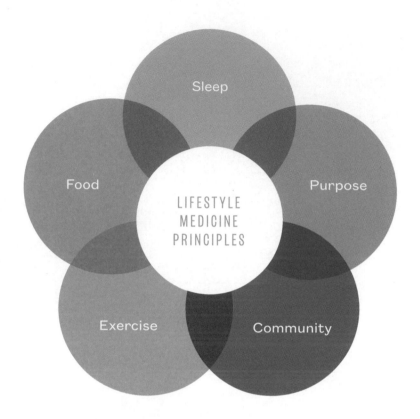

When we change our thinking from just reacting to and fighting off illness when it appears, to instead asking why it has occurred in the first place and what is its root cause, we can better understand how to use food as a way to build resilience to ill health and shift the prevailing medical paradigm from reactive to preventative medicine.

I also hope the 'food as medicine' encourages food retailers and industry to make healthy options the default, rather than marketing them as premium products we have to opt into. If we are serious about building the healthiest population possible, where chronic disease is a rarity, type 2 diabetes isn't an issue and heart disease affects fewer people, we need to start reforming our food systems and changing our food environment. And along with food, perhaps we could also reframe the way we consider exercise as medicine, sleep as medicine, connection, purpose and community as medicine. These are all tools that are just as important, and that we can utilise to create an environment that allows health to thrive rather than just stave off disease.

We are all hardwired for good health. There is simply nothing more elegant and beautiful than our perfectly functioning bodies, which we can better look after with healthy food and better lifestyle habits. Our evolutionary journey has equipped us with the biological machinery to thrive in the harshest of conditions and in this section you'll understand the inherent health systems that allow us to do so. I want to address how we can eat to beat illness and succinctly round up the science of 'food as medicine' as a way to motivate you to stick with the principles of healthy eating, exemplified by the 3-2-1 meals in this book. Armed with this knowledge I hope to nudge you into making healthier choices every day, to nourish your cells, reduce your risk of disease, optimise the function of your body and ultimately improve your wellbeing.

ANTIOXIDANTS AND FOOD

When healthcare practitioners, and those outside the profession, think of the impact of diet on human health, most of us think of the antioxidant capacity of fruits and vegetables. The traditional idea that antioxidants housed within citrus fruits, greens and other colourful vegetables are key to reducing the risk of disease is ingrained in most people's minds. A number of studies demonstrate that the more antioxidants one consumes through food, the more

antioxidant markers are found in the blood, and the markers associated with risk such as DNA damage and oxidised fats are lower. And while I agree that the antioxidants in food are able to neutralise pro-oxidant reactive species in cells and protect our DNA, which prevents a cascade of damage that could lead to harm, the story of antioxidants and food is largely over-simplified. Antioxidants alone cannot entirely explain the benefits of food.

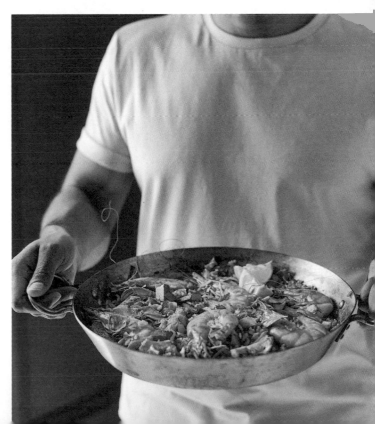

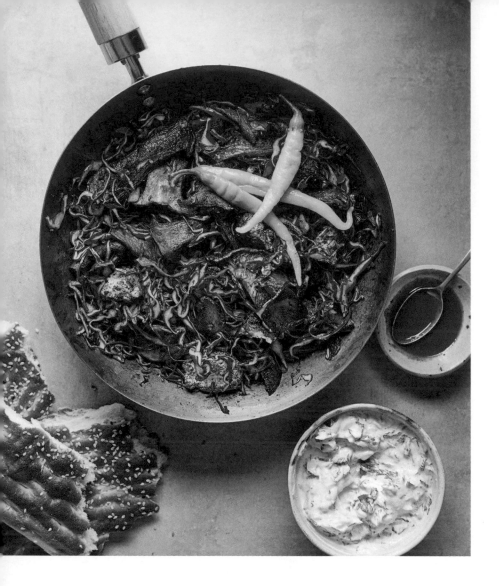

Fruits, vegetables, nuts and seeds contain a range of nutrients including minerals, vitamins, phytonutrients and many chemicals that are still yet to be discovered. These are perfectly arranged in a manner that allows them to act on multiple biological pathways synergistically. It is this feature of *whole* food that makes it distinct from a drug or a supplement that typically act on one pathway at a time.

The antioxidant theory scratches the surface of how what we eat can positively impact our physiology. Every time you take a bite of delicious wholesome food in the form of fruits and vegetables, the fibre positively impacts your gut microbe function, nutrients interact with your DNA to change the function of your cells and you are flooding your body with other plant chemicals that can positively impact your health. The ability of our food to impact our physiology is incredible and we all have the ability to engage these health systems.

INFLAMMATION

Inflammation is one of the most important and necessary functions of our body that has allowed us to adapt to our environment, heal wounds and fight infections. But the excess of inflammation in our bodies at a cellular level (related to high sugar consumption, poor sleep, insufficient exercise, stress and lack of adequate nutrients) is linked with a host of conditions including high blood pressure, diabetes and mental health problems.

Inflammation is meant to be a short lived, adaptive process that quickly resolves, but poor lifestyle and lack of proper nutrition leads to an imbalance of pro- and anti-inflammatory signals that can result in persistent low-grade inflammation (dubbed 'meta-inflammation' in the medical literature). It is this imbalance of inflammatory signals that a nutrient-dense diet with adequate portions of fruit, vegetables, nuts and seeds can help rectify.

Phytochemicals are produced by the plant as a form of insecticide to protect themselves from being eaten by pests, but these same chemicals have been found to impact processes in the human body related to inflammation. Polyphenols are types of plant chemicals found in brightly coloured fruit and vegetables that are potent inhibitors of inflammatory pathways. Other plant chemicals such as sulphur-containing compounds found in cruciferous vegetables contain potent anti-inflammatory properties that reduce oxidative stress as well as myriad others found in fruits and vegetables. The best way to obtain a dose of these inflammation balancing signals is to eat a variety of them and in appropriate doses, which is why 3-2-1 recipes are formulated to achieve this. Consuming a diverse range of colourful ingredients not only ensures a selection of different phytonutrients that can directly balance inflammation, but these foods also impact the microbes living in our gut. These microbes are important modulators of inflammation, among other things, that can improve our health immeasurably.

GUT MICROBIOTA

The gut microbiota refers to the diverse population of microbes that include viruses, fungi and bacteria found largely in the colon. Established in the first year of life, our gut microbiota co-evolves with the immune system and plays a role in the modulation of inflammation by decreasing systemic levels of inflammatory proteins and upregulating innate immune activity such as natural killer cells. In addition, they release nutrition from food, protect us from dangerous pathogens and the products of microbial fermentation create specialised short-chain fatty acids (such as acetate and butyrate), which provide energy sources for our digestive tract cells. There is simply no other area within nutritional medicine more fascinating at the moment than the study of this incredible population, which has far-reaching implications on the health of our brain, mental health, skin, immune system and more.

The suggestion that we can precisely manipulate the microbiota to alter its function using targeted foods, supplements, probiotics or other adjuncts is largely overestimated and warrants much further study. However, a number of studies have demonstrated that certain dietary patterns can nurture our microbes to help them best function. A dietary pattern (such as the Mediterranean diet) is a way of eating over an extended period of time, as opposed to a typical short-term 'diet' that is sustained for a few weeks or months but is often hard to maintain and can lead to 'yo-yoing'. The anti-inflammatory effect of the Mediterranean diet is well known and can in part be explained by significant changes in microbe gene

expression as well as biomarkers of inflammation.

Pulling the available research together, we also know that poor diet can rapidly shape the microbiota and likely cause intestinal inflammation and change the ability of microbes to appropriately function. A westernised diet, full of refined carbohydrates, excess sugar and lacking in essential micronutrients is universally bad for your microbes, and may increase your risk of inflammatory bowel disease, certain cancers and illnesses related to excess inflammation. Conversely, certain additions such as fruit fibres, pulses, beans and a diet comprised mostly of plants can have positive impacts on intestinal health and there are many mechanisms for how this can happen.

A pragmatic approach to improving the function and health of the gut microbiota would be to limit meat intake, increase intake of plant fibres, particularly from fruits and vegetables, and focus on diversity. All the 3-2-1 recipes are formulated with this in mind, and the principles of healthy eating will positively serve your microbes.

 DETOXIFICATION SYSTEMS

The word 'detox' is quite a loaded term. It conjures images of 'detox' teas,

We can improve our brain health, skin quality, mood and balance inflammation simultaneously, without having to count calories, reduce carbohydrates or follow any other restrictive guidelines.

supplements, cleanses and the barrage of overhyped products that lure people into a sense of feeling at risk unless they entertain some or all of these products. The commercial interests of companies have overstated the reality of what detoxification entails. Our bodies are actually incredibly self-sufficient when it comes to removing toxins from air, water, food and the natural waste products of normal metabolism, thanks to the action of our detoxification organs including the liver, lungs, skin and kidneys.

But there are ways to improve the capacity of our organs to deal with waste products beyond ensuring adequate hydration and exercise, and without having to spend exorbitant amounts on expensive supplements. For example, your liver is able to convert waste and toxin products into excretable compounds that are removed in faeces and urine, via enzymatic reactions. These reactions depend on co-factors that include

micronutrients and phytonutrients found in food such as colourful vegetables, citrus fruits and especially greens like broccoli.

A number of clinical studies have demonstrated an enhanced removal of air pollutants, measured by the amount found in subjects' urine, upon consuming more phytonutrients found in brassica vegetables, namely sulforaphane. A similar finding is true of the phytonutrient resveratrol found in wine, peanuts and grapes, and other cruciferous vegetables that contain indole-3-carbinol, which can upregulate enzymes in the liver responsible for detoxification. Studies looking at cells in lab conditions reveal that berries, spices such as ginger, and allium vegetables including onion and leek may also have the capacity to support our innate ability to detoxify. Research has also demonstrated that the accumulation of, and exposure to, environmental pollutants may in part be contributing to the plethora of chronic illnesses

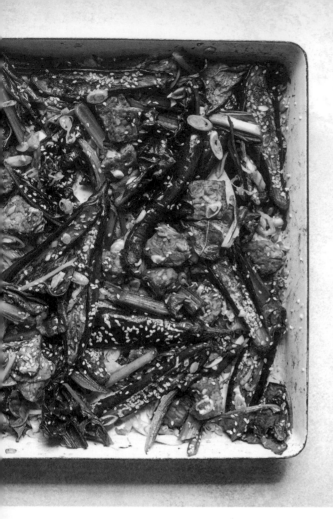

in the liver, these ingredients are also thought to increase detoxification by signalling specific genes and changing the function of the proteins they code for. This is yet another way in which food can impact our physiology.

 ## NUTRIGENOMICS

Genes are the molecular code that govern our physical and biological characteristics. Our genes are fixed, and these unique sequences inherited from both parents are unable to be changed by lifestyle. However, the expression and function of genes can be altered. The impact of nutrition on the expression of genes is known as the field of 'nutrigenomics' and describes how nutrient signals from the food we consume (which include vitamins, minerals, phytonutrients, amino acids, sugars and fatty acids) have the ability to change the genetic function of our cells. Quite literally, food is information and it has the capacity to interact with the very core of our existence, our DNA.

The ability of nutrients in food to communicate with our biology can sometimes happen via direct signals to cells that impact gene expression, and in other cases nutrients act as co-factors in metabolic processes that change gene function. Nutrients are also the building blocks for cellular function, without which cells are unable to

including obesity and heart disease. If true, the detoxification potential of a wholesome diet consisting of varied ingredients including herbs, spices, vegetables from the cruciferous and allium family may prove beneficial in the fight against illness.

Remember, it's not the food itself that detoxifies us, but rather the compounds in whole foods that support the normal detoxification processes of our body. Beyond upregulating certain enzymes function optimally. The more we learn about our individual differences in how we respond to different nutrient signals, the more targeted and personalised dietary advice we may be able to give that is specifically tailored to our genetic blueprint, a practice within nutrition called 'nutrigenetics'.

However, if we are able to get the basics right and grasp an understanding that our dietary pattern creates a plethora of signals that communicate with our cellular DNA, leading to an overall negative or positive outcome, a tailored nutrigenetic dietary profile is not always necessary. By following 3-2-1 recipes which focus on nutrient-dense ingredients, quality fats and whole foods, we can fulfil the requirements of a healthy diet that can positively influence our genetic expression to optimise cellular function and upregulate protective mechanisms that prevent illness.

PUTTING IT ALL TOGETHER

The beneficial characteristics of whole foods that positively interact with our body's health systems are designed to protect us from ill health and keep us thriving. The attributes of good food deliver incredible benefits to our longevity, immune system, cognition and mental health, to name a few, and this is why I'm so passionate about educating everybody on their ability to influence their own health for the better, by using their plate. Traditionally the impact of food is understated, and it is our responsibility to ensure that everybody understands the importance and impact of food to health. The benefits should not be sensationalised but, faced with the mammoth weight of evidence, we need to take our plates and our nutrition a lot more seriously than we have.

This isn't a plea to eat prescriptively or specifically for one attribute of food, whether it be its anti-inflammatory potential or its ability to enhance detoxification processes, but rather it should give you an understanding of how to eat to fuel our incredible internal ecosystem that already knows how to maintain itself. The purpose of all of my books are to get you in the kitchen and make it easier than ever to make changes that will have significant impacts on your health and hopefully the health of your family and loved ones, too.

Motivated by the incredible benefits of food, we can improve our brain health, skin quality, mood and balance inflammation simultaneously, without having to count calories, reduce carbohydrates or follow any other restrictive guidelines. The message is simple and clear, and the 3-2-1 recipes will make it easy to follow.

Should you fast?

The irony of talking about fasting in a cookbook is not lost on me. But, considering its popularity and the increase in interest from both nutrition experts and medical professionals alike (plus the number of times I'm asked about it by patients in clinic!), I think I should address the usefulness of fasting, as well as its pitfalls.

Built within our DNA is the incredible ability to survive the harshest of conditions. Our bodies are evolutionarily adapted to thrive during disease, harsh climates and especially during famine. Without this ability our species would have become extinct millions of years ago, so it was imperative for our genetic material to contain the code for switching on 'survival mode'. During the extensive hunter-gatherer period, before we developed the ability to settle and farm the land, our species would have had to deal with many situations where food was not readily available.

The production of food through better agricultural methods, which has led to the increased availability of food, is a relatively recent phenomenon spanning only the last 20,000 years. Despite how long that sounds, in the context of our evolutionary history it is a fraction of time. Fast forward to today's food landscape and we are privileged to have an abundance of produce from all corners of the globe and near 24-hour food provision. But this is coupled with a few cultural norms that may be detrimental to our health, considering what we now know about the benefits of fasting.

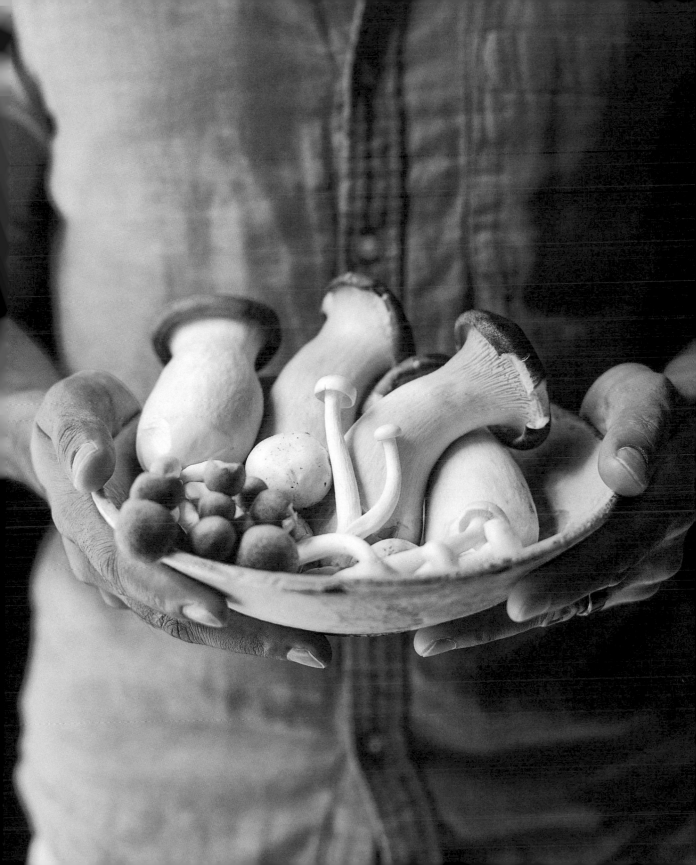

It is generally not acceptable that we should ever feel hungry. After all, there are starving people all over the globe suffering malnourishment who would relish the opportunity to have food, so why would you purposely endure circumstances that could do harm? The research, on the other hand, is shaking up our ingrained beliefs about 3 square meals a day, 2 snacks and a dessert at dinner, and the previous advice that we should feel satiated throughout our waking day, eating meals little and often.

Considering our evolutionary journey to the present day, there may actually be virtue in the absence of food, and experiencing hunger could be something we need to re-establish a relationship with. As controversial as it sounds, a fasting practice could help you live a longer, healthier life but it does not need to be as restrictive as a complete absence of food for days on end.

The practice of fasting has been hailed to bestow benefits to a number of different issues including glucose control in diabetes, autoimmune conditions and even cancer. Certain types of fasting can indeed improve sugar control in your blood, reduce inflammation and increase stress resistance, but what I've noticed in both the media and even the academic literature is confusion over what different fasting practices there are, how we define them and their relevance to individuals. 'Fasting' can be taken to mean a multitude of different practices: a very low-calorie diet over a few days a month; an 'eating window' of less than 10 hours a day; or even the complete absence of any nutrition except water for an extended period of time, which could be 24 hours or longer. Considering that the practice of fasting can be mean very different things, it's important to get the terminology correct right from the start.

Types of fasting

WATER FASTING

This is perhaps the most recognisable and extreme type of fasting. It involves the complete absence of nutrition apart from hydration with water, and can last anywhere between 24 hours and a week. Many faiths use fasting as an exercise during the observance of religious holidays, with the explanation that sacrificing food promotes interoception (an awareness and intuition of what's going on inside your body and mind) and perhaps improves one's connection with a higher entity. There are non-

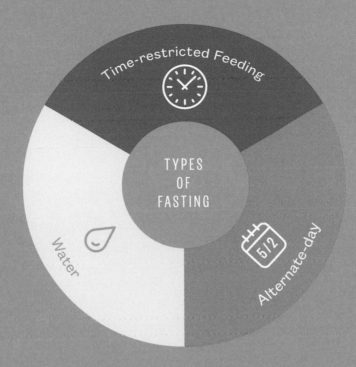

Time-restricted Feeding

TYPES
OF
FASTING

Water

Alternate-day

religious water fasting practices for health benefits, too, such as giving your gut a rest from digestive activity and accelerating the beneficial effects of fasting that I discuss below.

INTERMITTENT FASTING

Intermittent fasting (IF) is actually the most vague term for fasting and can be used to refer to multiple types of fasting including alternate-day fasting, fasting mimicking diets and time-restricted feeding (TRF).

TIME-RESTRICTED FEEDING

Perhaps thought of as the new kid on the block, time-restricted feeding (TRF) is generally accepted to mean not eating food for anywhere between 12 and 18 hours in a 24-hour period, where there is no change to the calorie content of your daily intake. For example, an 18:6 regimen is where you allow yourself the opportunity to eat only within 6 hours of your day and typically this can mean starting an eating window at 12pm and having your last meal before 6pm, with no snacking in between. But, it can also be as gentle as a 12:12 regimen, where you stop eating at 8pm in the evening if you had breakfast at 8am.

ALTERNATE-DAY FASTING

Intermittent fasting can also refer to alternate-day fasting (ADF), and this is where there is a lot of confusion in both the evidence base and the media. The most popular alternate day fasting method is the 5:2 diet, where a normal calorie-controlled diet is consumed for 5 days and a significantly reduced calorie diet (less than 800 calories per 24 hours) is consumed for the remaining 2 days. But there are variations of this such as Professor Valter Longo's 'Fasting Mimicking Diet' (FMD), which is a continuous 5-day, sub 500-calorie regimen usually practiced once a month or every other month. The exciting premise of FMD is that it has been used in both animal and human studies as an adjunct to chemotherapy in cancer patients and immune suppressant therapy in people with autoimmune conditions with some encouraging early results. In addition, alternate-day fasting can also refer to a complete water fast for 24 hours or longer.

From the descriptions of these various types of fasting, I hope you can understand why the term 'fasting' can be exceptionally vague and misleading.

It's almost equivalent to declaring that you 'eat food' when somebody asks about your diet. The fact is everybody fasts. When we are asleep we are essentially fasting, so in a sense we are always 'intermittently fasting'. But the degree to which we extend the fasting window, or reduce total energy consumption on a given day, may yield completely different outcomes. Who benefits from which type of fasting practice is still the frustratingly difficult unanswered question, but on a more positive note, we are learning more about the potential mechanisms of how fasting works.

How fasting works

Our genetic material contains the code to alter our metabolism, change inflammation pathways and adjust cell signalling, and this beautifully coordinated effort coalesces to increase resilience and thus survival in times of distress. Along with exercise, cold water therapy and sleep, fasting practices have been shown to harness this incredible machinery that lives within all of us and may extend both healthspan as well as longevity. While we don't completely know what mechanisms are responsible for the benefits, lab studies and human trials have given us some insight into the potential pathways.

METABOLIC SWITCHING

During periods when food is not consumed, your body preferentially uses glucose in your liver, where it is stored in a form called glycogen. Once those stores are used up, a metabolic switch is triggered, which encourages your body to use fats and ketones for fuel instead of sugar (these are found in your fat cells and liver). Adapting to the use of fats and ketones, instead of sugars found in food, upregulates a number of pathways that improve the efficiency of energy generation in your cells by organelles called mitochondria and increases resilience to stress.

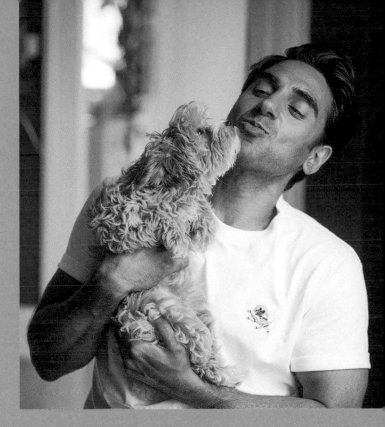

KETONE PRODUCTION

Most of us produce small amounts of ketones when waking up from sleep because as our glucose levels fall during our overnight 'fast' and your body starts breaking down fats and producing ketones in the liver to maintain cellular energy. Ketone production is increased during longer periods without food, and it turns out ketones are more than just another source of fuel for your cells: ketones are signalling molecules that change the expression of your genes – they can reduce inflammation and may even have beneficial effects on the function of brain cells specifically.

INFLAMMATION

The production of ketones, reduction in glucose, as well as dampening insulin production during fasting may suppress something called the inflammasome, a component of our immune system that, when it's at high levels, is linked to obesity-related diseases and type 2 diabetes. Fasting is also associated with reduced circulating pro-inflammatory molecules including homocysteine, interleukins (such as IL-6) and C-reactive protein (CRP) that can contribute to cardiovascular disease and types of dementia. During fasting, fat cells release a protein called adiponectin that can prevent arterial blockages that cause heart attacks by reducing the inflammation within the walls of coronary vessels.

NUTRIENT SENSING AND AUTOPHAGY

Our cells have developed incredible capabilities to sense the nutrient status of our body and adapt their functions accordingly. In a fasted state where both protein and glucose levels are low, the body upregulates 'nutrient sensing genes' that act to stimulate the process of autophagy. Autophagy is a highly regulated and coordinated process of recycling components from cells that are old or damaged. These components are broken down into their basic structures like fatty acids from fats and amino acids from protein, ready to make brand new cells when the body is fuelled again with nutrition. This self-preservation mechanism of creating new cells while clearing older or dysfunctional ones, along with a milieu of other processes, are potential explanations as to why fasting appears to enhance longevity and increase healthspan. We have only touched the surface on how autophagy could potentially reduce the risk of cancer and Alzheimer's, but the evolving science may eventually show it to be an effective complementary tool in the fight against disease.

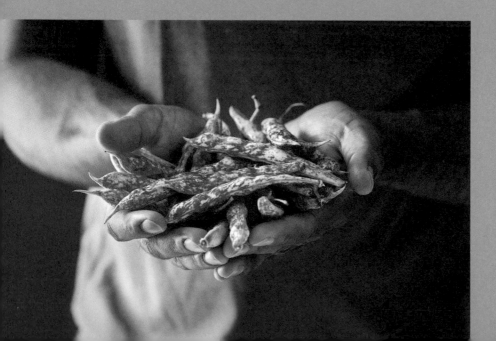

USES

Overall, fasting seems to confer health benefits to a greater extent than can be attributed just to a reduction in calorie intake. Considering the mechanistic pathways that are switched on through different forms of fasting and its impact (particularly on inflammation and autophagy) there are many potential uses for fasting as a clinical tool, in tackling obesity, Alzheimer's, autoimmune conditions, hypertension, type 1 and 2 diabetes as well as a potential use alongside cancer therapy.

SO SHOULD YOU?

I don't want this to sound like a big advert for fasting because within this exercise are potential pitfalls. Fasting may increase gut permeability that can lead to digestive problems, it could lead to psychological stress, there may be issues with medication and fasting can also have a negative impact on medical problems such as thyroid conditions as well as worsening or contributing to eating disorders. It's not a black and white subject. The 'dose' of fasting, what type, the regularity of fasts and whether we should 'cycle' fasting periods are all topics open for discussion and as of yet it is hard to match the types of fasting to different patient groups.

Time-restricted feeding, on the other hand, is less rigid than other forms of fasting and still allows you to eat delicious meals that you'll find in this book, without worrying about counting calories or forcing yourself to avoid all food for days at a time. The simple exercise of eating in a defined window of 10–11 hours is a gentle method of potentially improving your overall health and avoiding unnecessary late-night snacks. This is why one of my principles is 'eating in time', which refers to ensuring your meals are eaten in this rough time period every day. Practically, this could mean eating breakfast at 9am and eating dinner before 7pm, which is achievable for many of us. This method of eating makes use of your inbuilt machinery to improve sugar control, activate longevity genes, upregulate autophagy and enhance insulin sensitivity without unnecessarily starving yourself.

And so to respond to the question 'should you fast?': quite honestly, I have no idea. And I think we are a while away from determining which method of fasting is more effective and suited to different people based on age, convenience and genetic history. But defining your eating window using TRF is a simple hack that has been shown to have health benefits. I would regard it as safe, and it is an approach to eating I personally follow and recommend. Perhaps give it a try during the '3-2-1 week kickstarter' and see how you feel.

How to 3-2-1

Over the last decade of my medical career I've spoken to and treated thousands of patients and learnt from hundreds of medical colleagues. In addition to my clinical practice, since launching The Doctor's Kitchen, I have gained insight from tens of thousands of people across the globe who want to learn more about food and lifestyle medicine. Together, this varied experience has led me to understand that informing people about the power of food and lifestyle choices alone is simply not enough.

In my previous two books I hammered home some core facts about the beauty of food and the impact of eating well on our health, and took readers on a journey through the science of food as medicine. In my last book I also highlighted in each chapter the large body of evidence that specifically covers how food can be used to heighten cognitive performance, prevent heart disease, improve skin quality and even help manage mental health problems.

But, despite recognising and understanding how pivotal nutrition is for preventing disease and optimising health, people from all walks of life across the globe still struggle to maintain the motivation and ability to eat well every day. I've come to realise that in addition to educating, I need to focus on the pain points and barriers to healthy living, so I can provide guidance on how to navigate common obstacles and make the process of looking after your wellbeing as frictionless

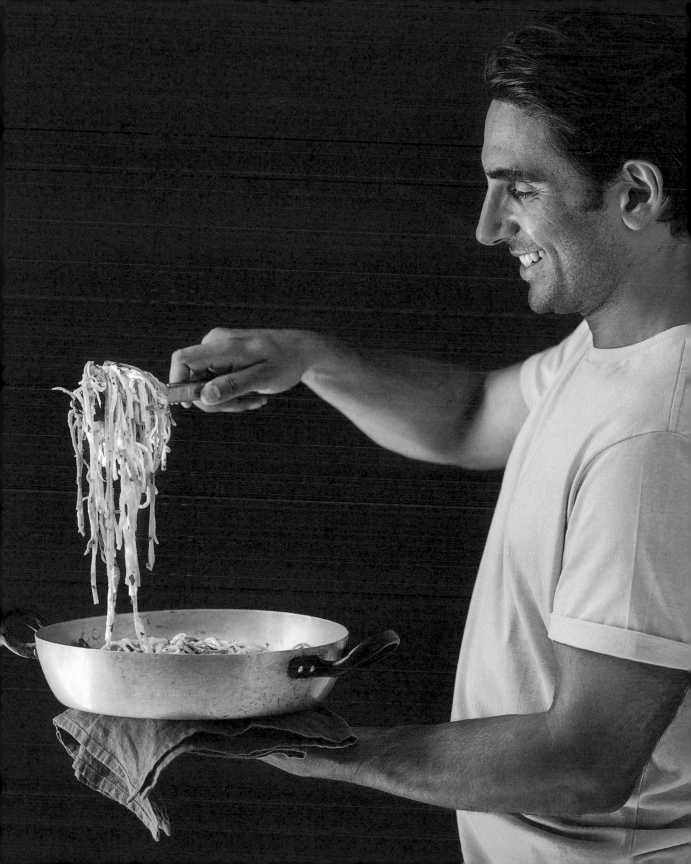

as possible. Once we understand why we struggle to maintain healthy eating in the long term, we can work to ensure we hit our health objectives consistently and take back control of our wellbeing.

Taking control

In writing this book, answering these two questions has been key:

1   How do I motivate you to start eating well?

2   How do I create a framework for you to maintain eating well for life?

By virtue of picking up this book I'm sure you are already motivated to start making changes, or perhaps maintain the ones you've already made. If not, I hope that after reading the first few chapters I've convinced you that consistently eating a plant-focused diet is associated with a number of health benefits and now is the time to start.

The key word in all of this is 'consistency'. Your diet will ebb and flow with the changing course of your week or month which, in a nutshell, is why restrictive diets tend not to work in the long run. Think about what you eat over the long term rather than short term. It's not each individual meal choice that affects our health, it's our habits over a long time period. It is totally fine and absolutely healthy to indulge on occasion, and allow yourself to be flexible with your eating habits. You just need to ensure that the vast majority of your meals are the types that feed your health rather than risk it.

This book is here to guide you to make healthy meals the norm, and the 3-2-1 recipes are geared towards helping you maintain your journey by reducing all the common barriers and allowing you to kickstart healthy eating.

Once we understand why we struggle to maintain healthy eating in the long term, we can work to ensure we hit our health objectives consistently.

3-2-1 principles

In all my books the principles of healthy eating have remained the same. Considering the headlines over the last decade you may think that my nutritional stance should have swayed from low carb, to vegan, then paleo and perhaps back to 100 per cent plant-based, but as a doctor I choose not ride the wave of populism, nor do I pander to current trends. I am guided by the evidence.

This is why I have held to the same core messages regarding healthy eating: plant focused, lots of fibre, plenty of colourful vegetables, eating whole and eating within a defined window of time (see page 38 for more on fasting).

Looking at all the evidence available to us, it is clear that this continues to be the way we should be eating, and as a responsible, credible physician with an interest in nutrition, this is why I promote it. You can rest assured I have done the hard work of analysing the studies for you and now you can enjoy delicious recipes in the knowledge that they will certainly be good for you.

ACCESSIBLE, AFFORDABLE AND DELICIOUS

The most incredible, nutrient-dense ingredients we all have access to are often the cheapest on the shelf. What limits our ability to use them is this idea that we're not great cooks and that we lack culinary creativity, as well as a belief that these ingredients are expensive. These are myths. The ingredients highlighted in each recipe in this book are 'normal' ingredients that contain a powerful orchestra of nutrients that can deliver health benefits.

Everything from a simple carrot to your humble apple deserves the 'superfood' status traditionally reserved for more expensive items. These everyday, affordable and accessible ingredients are key to good health. What's more, eating plates of a variety of colourful plants is the easiest way to contribute towards our wellbeing, and it's what makes the 3-2-1 recipes in this book appear so vibrant. It is the amount and variety of ingredients we need to focus on, rather than a prescriptive list of overpriced or specific ingredients.

You may find that eating the 3-2-1 way even reduces your weekly food bill, too. Health isn't just for the financially privileged or those who have more time in their day – it can be accessible to everyone and no more expensive than the average household can afford.

DIVERSITY IS THE GOAL

Every micronutrient is inextricably linked to another, so supplementing individual micronutrients in isolation or eating a limited range of 'superfoods' every week is unlikely to provide the wholesome benefits to your inner ecosystem of microbes largely living in your gut (more on this on page 33). This ecosystem actually thrives on diversity: variety is king, and diversifying what you eat on a weekly basis is actually one of the best health strategies I could recommend. What this means in practical terms is experimenting with new vegetables on a weekly basis, trying what's in season and diversifying your culinary habits with new recipes that 3-2-1 will help you achieve.

COOKING FROM SCRATCH IS KEY

I can outline any number of scientific observations that demonstrate the benefits of cooking from scratch at least once a day, not least the better nutrient profile of ingredients and the enhanced absorption of nutrients when meals are cooked with fresh produce. I believe that cooking is

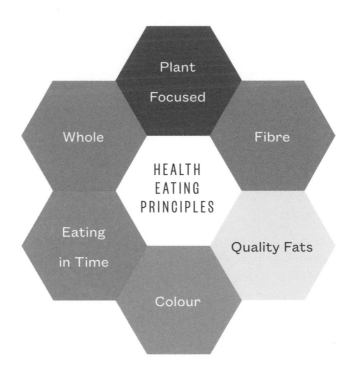

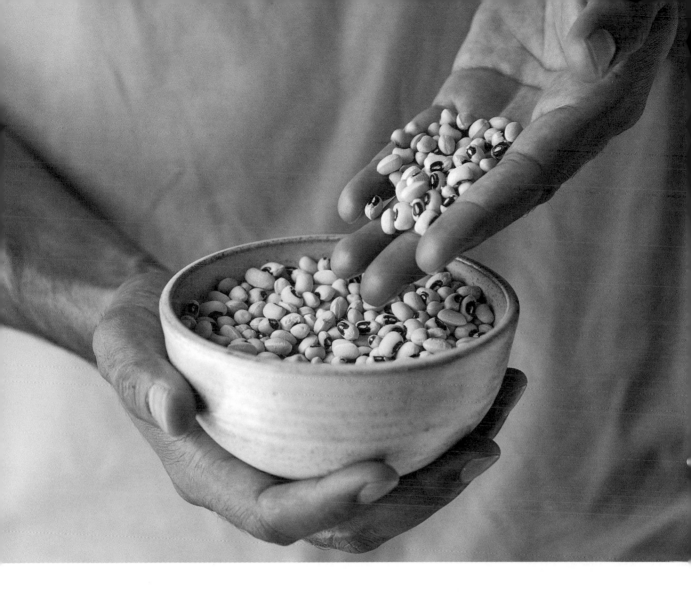

fundamental to our existence. It is part of our evolutionary process to have been sitting around a heat source, or foraging for plants, then sharing food with our family and community. The additional intangible benefits of this communal aspect of eating are another reason I want to persuade you to cook

from scratch at least once a day. An investment of as little as 10 minutes of mental effort and food preparation is all you need, and if you don't believe me then I challenge you to try the '3-2-1 week kickstarter' on the following page that will launch your healthy eating journey.

The 3-2-1 week kickstarter

This 'kickstarter' invites you to give yourself the opportunity to adopt this new way of cooking and owning your kitchen. It will change your ability to cook and look after your health every day using food. For one week you will be a 3-2-1 cook.

START A HEALTHY EATING HABIT

We easily adopt so many behaviours that negatively influence how we view ourselves, to the detriment of forming habits that benefit our wellbeing. If we don't believe that we can easily learn how to cook, or that we lack the time, the culinary creativity or the ability to create food that looks and tastes delicious every day, then that is what our reality becomes. We won't allow ourselves to grow into forming new habits unless we first believe that we can achieve them. I had this dismissive mindset before I got ill with a medical condition that forced me to make time for self care: 'I'm too busy to cook. I can't afford the ingredients. I'm too tired.'

These were all completely, reasonable excuses for a new junior doctor, considering I had just started a demanding hospital job characterised by night shifts, gruelling long-hour days and the stresses of learning new critical skills. And they still are absolutely legitimate reasons for a lot of us in similarly demanding lifestyles, whether that be work pressures, family commitments or a combination of both. But, when I was forced to make time for self care, as a result of an unusual heart condition I developed three months into starting work as a doctor, I realised the excuses I made were the product of my inability to find solutions to an important problem. And my poor diet and lifestyle was in part related to my heart condition that I needed to address. I hear the same excuses I used to tell myself in clinic from patients and medical colleagues alike, which is exactly how and why this book has come about. The barriers to eating well every day are not as high as we perceive them to be, and this chapter demonstrates how easy it can be to consistently eat well, with just a few minutes of prep per meal.

With that in mind, the 'kickstarter' outlines how you can make breakfast, lunch and dinner in just 15 minutes of prep time a day.

I hope these recipes also allow you the space to learn how to enjoy other aspects of lifestyle medicine such as mindfulness and movement that are just as important as cooking, too.

The 15-minute mealtime promise is painstakingly simple:

5 minutes of prep for breakfast and 10 minutes prep for dinner and lunch. Some days you'll already have breakfast made so can spend a little more time on dinner. Each meal has 2 servings, so you can use the leftovers for the next day.

If you want to do the kickstarter for 2 people, just double the ingredients.

It's that straightforward.

Health is something you practice daily and the collection of meals you consume will guide you on that journey. Try these one-pan meals for a week that take the effort out of cooking and put the health and enjoyment back in, and I guarantee it will kickstart a habit for life.

And whenever you feel like you need a kickstart you can add different recipes to this list to help you stay on track.

Just give me 15 minutes every day for a week and I will turn you into a Doctor's Kitchen cook!

	SUNDAY	MONDAY	TUESDAY	WEDNESDAY
	Total prep time 10 mins	Total prep time 10 mins	Total prep time 5 mins	Total prep time 10 mins
MORNING		COOK Fig and Blackberry Porridge (page 60)	LEFTOVERS Fig and Blackberry Porridge	COOK Peach and Cardamom Baked Oats (page 64)
LUNCH		LEFTOVERS Massaman Cauliflower	LEFTOVERS Coconut Yellow Dhal with Tamarind and Curry Leaves	LEFTOVERS Red Bean Giouvetsi
EVENING	COOK Massaman Cauliflower (page 134)	COOK Coconut Yellow Dhal with Tamarind and Curry Leaves (page 184)	COOK Red Bean Giouvetsi (page 222)	COOK Mango Pickle and Squash Curry (page 186)

THURSDAY	FRIDAY	SATURDAY	SUNDAY
Total prep time 15 mins	Total prep time 15 mins	Total prep time 10 mins	Total prep time 15 mins

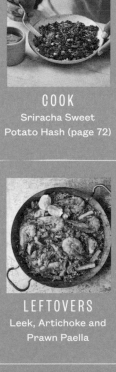	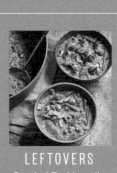	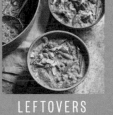	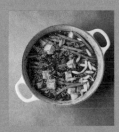
LEFTOVERS	**COOK**	**LEFTOVERS**	**COOK**
Peach and Cardamom Baked Oats	Sriracha Sweet Potato Hash (page 72)	Sriracha Sweet Potato Hash	Huevos Rancheros (page 82)

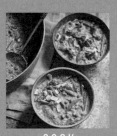		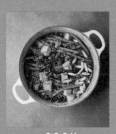	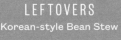
LEFTOVERS	**LEFTOVERS**	**LEFTOVERS**	**LEFTOVERS**
Mango Pickle and Squash Curry	Leek, Artichoke and Prawn Paella	Sambal Red Lentils	Korean-style Bean Stew

COOK	**COOK**	**COOK**	
Leek, Artichoke and Prawn Paella (page 130)	Sambal Red Lentils (page 188)	Korean-style Bean Stew (page 220)	

Everyday hero foods

Armed with this new knowledge, I hope you're just as enthusiastic as me about eating a diverse range of these wonderful ingredients. Wholesome foods in their natural unprocessed state are absolutely incredible. They contain an orchestra of chemicals that are perfectly arranged to provide nourishment to our bodies when we consume them. Below is a collection of some of the '3' portions of fruits, vegetables, nuts and seeds used in the recipes and an example of their nutritional content. Remember, each ingredient is more than the sum of the plant chemicals, vitamins and minerals it contains, and these are just reminders of how beautiful and complex our humble everyday ingredients are.

 NUTS
Protein and minerals

 SEEDS
Protein and minerals

 BEANS
Plant sterols

 CHICKPEAS
Fibre and protein

 LENTILS
Fibre and protein

 APPLES
Quercetin

 BANANAS
Pectin fibre

 BLACKBERRIES
Anthocyanins

 BLUEBERRIES
Anthocyanins

 FIGS
Soluble fibre

 JACKFRUIT
Fibre

 MANGOES
Carotenoids

 PEACHES
Flavanols

 PEARS
Flavanols

 PINEAPPLES
Bromelain

 POMELOS
Flavonoids

ARTICHOKES
Prebiotic fibres

ASPARAGUS
Phenolic compounds

AVOCADOS
Magnesium

AUBERGINES
Nasunin

BEANS (GREEN/ RUNNER)
Folate

BEANSPROUTS
Vitamin C

BEETROOTS
Betalain

BROAD BEANS
Iron

BROCCOLI
Sulforaphane

BRUSSELS SPROUTS
Glucosinolates

CABBAGE (RED/ WHITE/CHINESE/ SAVOY)
Isothiocyanates

CARROTS
Carotenoids

CAULIFLOWER
Brassica vegetables

CELERIAC
Flavonoids

CELERY
Apigenin

COURGETTES
Potassium

CUCUMBERS
Triterpenes

FENNEL
Kaempferol

KALE/CAVOLO NERO/ SPRING GREENS
B vitamins

KIMCHI
Probiotic

LEEKS
Prebiotic fibre

LETTUCE
Vitamin C

MANGETOUT
Potassium

MUSHROOMS
Ergothioneine

ONIONS
Allicin

PAK CHOI
Glucosinolates

PARSNIPS
Fibre

PEA SHOOTS
Vitamin C

PEAS
Fibre and protein

PEPPERS
Vitamin C

RADICCHIO
Luteolin

RADISHES
Sulforaphane

ROCKET
Sulphur compounds

SPINACH
Folate

SPRING ONIONS
Allicin

SQUASH/PUMPKIN
Zeaxanthin and lutein

SUGAR SNAP PEAS
Iron

SWEETCORN
Carotenoids

SWEET POTATOES
Beta carotene

SWISS CHARD
Vitamin K

TOMATOES
Lycopene

WATER CHESTNUTS
Fibre

WATERCRESS
Zeaxanthin and lutein

CHICORY
Prebiotic fibre

Oats

An intense-coloured porridge with jammy figs and richness from the nut butter.

Fig and Blackberry Porridge

1 Lightly toast the oats, hemp seed (if using) and almonds in a dry medium saucepan over a low heat for 2–3 minutes. Pick out the almonds and save them to garnish.

2 Add the nut milk, blackberries, most of the figs, almond butter and salt. Then cook, stirring, for 10 minutes, adding a little more milk if it thickens too much.

3 Slice the toasted almonds. Spoon the porridge into two bowls and top with the remaining figs and the toasted sliced almonds, and drizzle with the maple syrup or honey.

PREP 5 MINS/COOK 15 MINS

100g porridge oats
50g shelled hemp seed (optional)
30g almonds
500ml nut milk, plus extra if needed
160g frozen or fresh blackberries
160g figs (about 4), sliced into wedges
30g smooth almond butter
pinch of salt
1 tbsp maple syrup or honey

Variation

Try using different fruits such as passionfruit, frozen cherries or mixed summer berries.

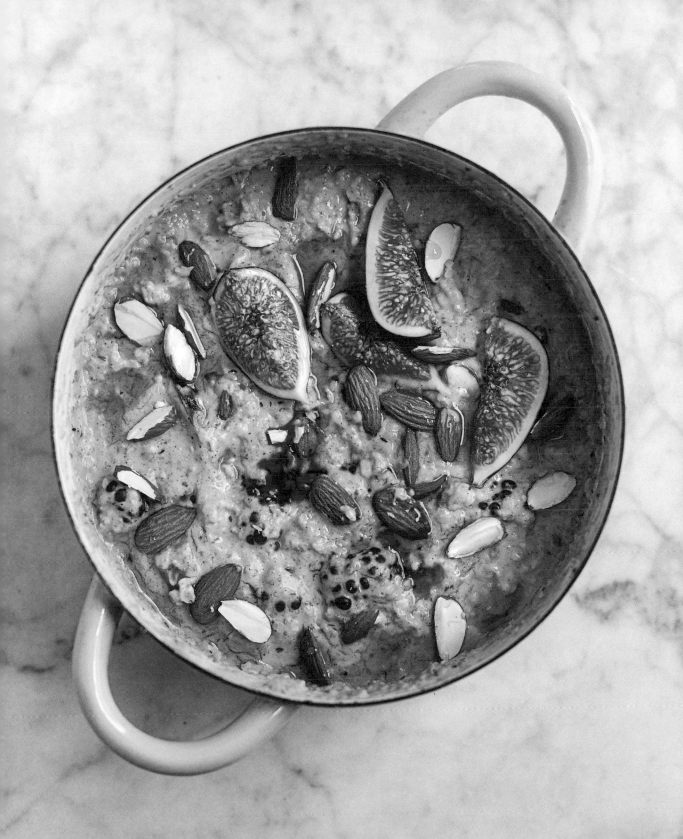

This comforting dish has an indulgent flavour from the coconut flakes, which pairs beautifully with fresh blueberries.

Pear, Blueberry and Coconut Baked Oats

1 Preheat the oven to 190°C/170°C fan/gas 5.

2 Mix the oats, hemp seed (if using) and most of the coconut and nuts in a 1–1.2-litre ovenproof dish. Stir in the nut milk, salt and fruit.

3 Bake in the oven for 15 minutes until the oats are creamy and most of the milk has been absorbed.

4 Serve in bowls with a drizzle of maple syrup and almond butter, and scatter with the reserved coconut and pistachios.

PREP 5 MINS/COOK 15 MINS

100g porridge oats
50g shelled hemp seed (optional)
30g coconut flakes
60g shelled, unsalted pistachios, roughly sliced
500ml nut milk
pinch of salt
160g peeled and cored pear (about 1 pear), sliced
160g blueberries
1 tbsp maple syrup
2 tbsp smooth almond butter

Variation

You can use apples instead of pears if you prefer.

A delightful dish with a mixture of natural sweetness from the stone fruit plus intense colour from the pistachios.

Mango and Pomegranate Porridge

1 Toast the oats, hemp seed (if using) and pistachios in a dry medium saucepan over a low heat for 2–3 minutes until they start to take on a little colour. Pick out a few toasted pistachios to garnish.

2 Stir in the milk, star anise, salt, frozen mango and sliced stone fruit. Cook, stirring, for 10 minutes, adding a little more milk if it starts to thicken too much.

3 Spoon into two bowls, drizzle with maple syrup and scatter with the pomegranate seeds and the toasted pistachios.

PREP 5 MINS/COOK 15 MINS

100g porridge oats
50g shelled hemp seed (optional)
60g shelled, unsalted pistachios, sliced
500ml nut milk, plus extra if needed
1 star anise
pinch of salt
160g frozen diced mango
160g destoned fresh stone fruit (such as peach, nectarine or plum), sliced
1 tbsp maple syrup
50g pomegranate seeds

Cook's tip

If you can find them, buy the ready-nibbed pistachios from Middle Eastern shops that have been skinned and are a fabulous green colour.

Variation

Try this dish with 3 lightly bashed cardamom pods instead of star anise (remember to remove before serving).

Baking oats in the oven is a revelation to me. I sometimes serve this simple dish warm, with ice cream, as a dessert.

Peach and Cardamom Baked Oats

1 Preheat the oven to 190°C/170°C fan/gas 5.

2 Mix the oats, hemp seed (if using) and most of the nuts in a 1–1.2-litre ovenproof dish. Stir in the nut milk, cardamom pods and salt. Add the mashed and sliced banana and the sliced peach and stir together.

3 Bake in the oven for 15 minutes until the oats are creamy and most of the milk has been absorbed.

4 Remove from the oven, discard the cardamom pods, then serve in bowls, drizzled with maple syrup and scattered with the remaining nuts.

Cook's tip

You can use a generous pinch of ground cardamom instead of cardamom pods.

PREP 5 MINS/COOK 15 MINS

100g porridge oats
50g shelled hemp seed (optional)
60g hazelnuts, roughly chopped
500ml nut milk
3 cardamom pods, cracked open
pinch of salt
160g peeled bananas (about 2), 1 mashed and 1 sliced
160g destoned fresh peach (about 1), sliced
1 tbsp maple syrup

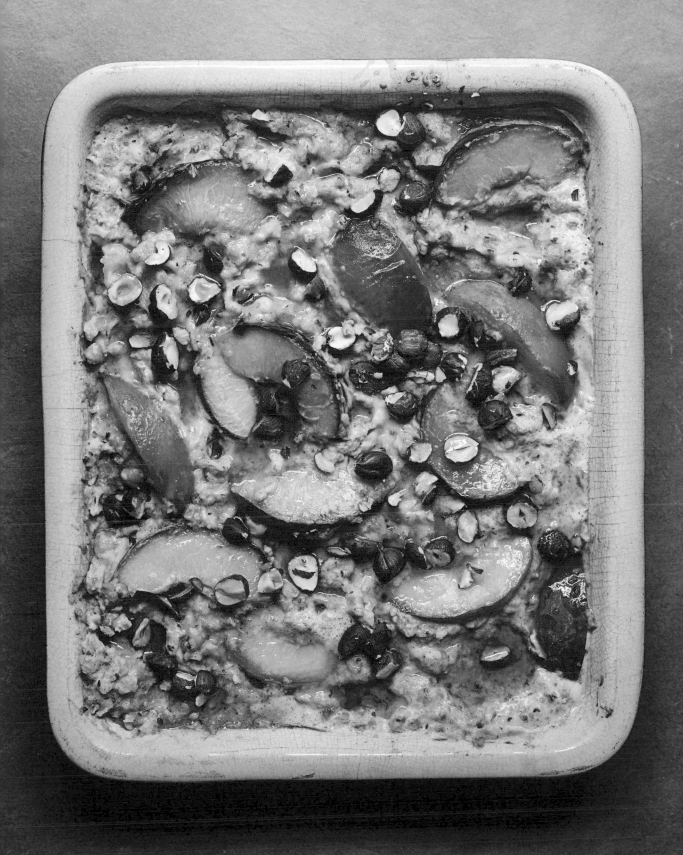

Overnight oats are my saviour for busy weeks, and this simply flavoured recipe is one of my favourites. The chia seeds are optional, but using them gives the soaked oats a jelly-like texture that makes the dish lighter.

Pistachio and Pear Overnight Oats

1 Mix together the oats, chia seeds (if using) and cardamom in a 500ml serving glass or jar.

2 Dollop the yoghurt on top, then add the nut milk, grated pear and pistachios. Mix well, cover and chill overnight.

3 In the morning, uncover and serve into two bowls.

4 Top each bowl with another dollop of yoghurt, the blueberries and the rest of the pistachios. Drizzle with honey or maple syrup and serve.

PREP 5 MINS

100g porridge oats

1 tbsp chia seeds (optional)

¼ tsp ground cardamom

4 tbsp Greek yoghurt, plus 2 tbsp extra to serve

120ml nut milk

160g grated pear (about 1 pear)

60g shelled, unsalted pistachios, chopped, plus 10g extra to serve

160g blueberries

1 tbsp honey or maple syrup, for drizzling

The pairing of the classic winter flavours of allspice and cinnamon with carrot is one of my favourite combinations, and it works wonderfully in this simple overnight oats recipe.

Cinnamon Apple and Carrot Overnight Oats

1 Mix together the oats, ground almonds and spices in a 500ml serving glass or storage jar.

2 Add the nut milk, grated apple and carrot. Mix well, cover and chill overnight.

3 In the morning, uncover and serve into two bowls.

4 Top each bowl with the yoghurt, drizzle with the honey or maple syrup and serve.

PREP TIME 5 MINUTES

100g porridge oats
60g ground almonds
pinch of ground allspice
¼ tsp ground cinnamon
175ml nut milk
160g apple (1–2 apples), grated
160g carrots (1 large or 2 small), grated

TO SERVE
3 tbsp Greek yoghurt
1 tbsp honey or maple syrup

Breakfast and Brunch

This dish reminds me of breakfast as a child growing up in an Indian household. Hot and spicy breakfast dishes sprinkled with garam masala and brimming with vegetables were the norm, and you will love this rapid version of one of my favourites.

Masala One-pan Breakfast

1 Toast the sesame seeds in a dry frying pan over a low heat for a minute until just golden, then scoop out of the pan and set aside.

2 Add the oil or ghee to the pan, increase the heat to medium and fry the onion gently for 10 minutes until softened, then add the cumin seeds and fry for a minute more.

3 Add the kale and a splash of water (about 50ml), cover and steam for 1–2 minutes until the kale is just tender and a little bit juicy.

4 Add the chickpeas, peas and garam masala, season well with salt and pepper and cook, uncovered, for 2–3 minutes, then remove from the heat.

5 Stir in the lemon juice and serve with a dollop of yoghurt, scattered with the toasted sesame seeds, chilli flakes and coriander leaves.

PREP 10 MINS/COOK 15 MINS

1 tbsp sesame seeds
2 tbsp coconut oil or ghee
120g onion (about 1 small), thinly sliced
2 tsp cumin seeds
160g trimmed kale, roughly sliced
400g tin chickpeas, drained and rinsed
160g frozen peas
1 tsp garam masala
squeeze of lemon juice
sea salt and freshly ground black pepper

TO SERVE
2–3 tbsp coconut yoghurt
pinch of dried chilli flakes
10g fresh coriander leaves

A classic recipe of spicy beans. I still love beans on toast, and with the right ingredients it can be nostalgic, flavourful and absolutely healthy. In fact, this recipe packs 4 portions of your 5-a-day per serving.

Spicy Baked Beans

1 Heat the oil in a sauté pan over a low to medium heat, add the shallots and fry gently for about 2–3 minutes until slightly softened. Add the garlic, thyme and harissa paste and fry for a minute or two more.

2 Add the passata, vinegar and black treacle (if using), season with salt and pepper and simmer gently for 2 minutes.

3 Add the red peppers and beans and cook for another 3–4 minutes until the sauce has reduced and the beans are coated all over.

4 Remove from the heat, stir through the spinach and allow to wilt, then fold in the parsley and serve on sourdough toast.

PREP 5 MINS/COOK 15 MINS

2 tbsp extra-virgin olive oil
90g banana shallot (about 1), finely chopped
2 garlic cloves, grated
4 or 5 sprigs of thyme
1 tbsp harissa paste
200g passata
1 tsp red wine vinegar
1 tbsp black treacle (optional)
160g roasted red peppers from a jar, sliced
400g tin white beans, drained and rinsed
160g baby leaf spinach, roughly chopped
20g fresh flat-leaf parsley, chopped
sea salt and freshly ground black pepper
toasted sourdough bread, to serve

Sriracha and sweet potato is one of my favourite flavour combinations. The natural sweetness of the potato and the hits of fiery flavour from the red sauce are beautiful together.

Sriracha Sweet Potato Hash

1 Heat the oil in a pan over a low heat, add the sweet potato and onion and fry, covered, for 6–8 minutes until the potato is just tender.

2 Uncover, and lightly mash with a fork to create some crispy edges.

3 Add the garlic and sriracha and fry for a minute, then add the sweetcorn. Spread in an even layer in the pan and fry over a medium heat, without stirring, for a good 4–5 minutes, to allow a bit of a crusty layer to form on the bottom.

4 Add the cavolo nero to the pan, stir, season with salt and pepper, cover and cook for 2–3 minutes until the greens are wilted and just cooked.

5 Remove from the heat and serve with the dill and extra sriracha.

PREP 10–15 MINS/COOK 15 MINS

2 tbsp extra-virgin olive oil

160g purple (or orange) sweet potatoes, cut into 1.5cm cubes

160g red onion (about 1 medium), thinly sliced

2 garlic cloves, grated

1 tbsp sriracha, plus extra for drizzling

120g sweetcorn kernels (fresh or frozen)

160g trimmed cavolo nero, shredded

sea salt and freshly ground black pepper

10g fresh dill, chopped, to serve

Cook's tip

Sriracha is a type of chilli sauce frequently used in Thai and other Asian dishes, but you could use any chilli sauce or a pinch of dried chilli flakes and a dash of rice vinegar or distilled malt vinegar.

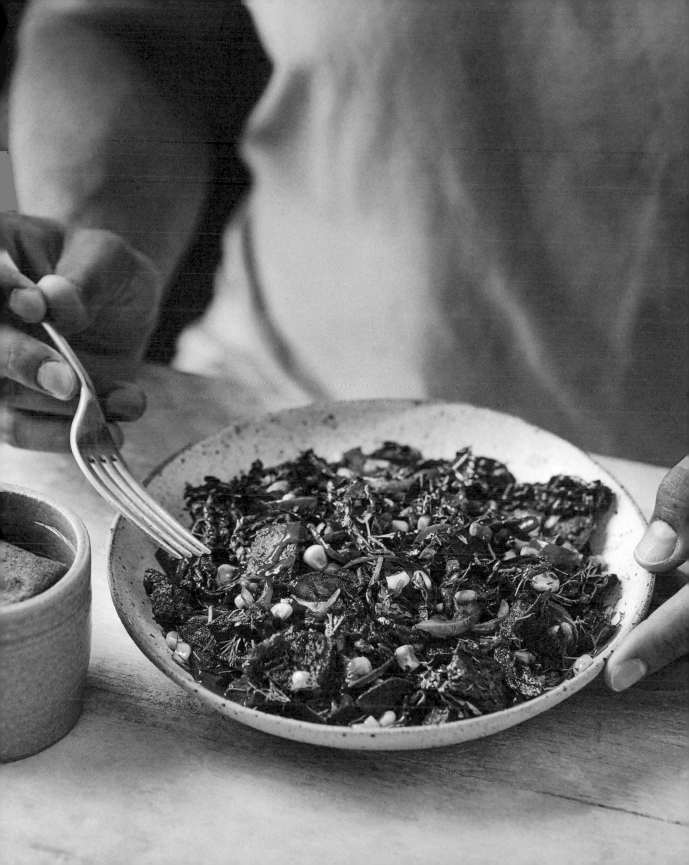

This recipe uses a jolly mixture of Middle Eastern ingredients to create something unique that also makes good use of seasonal spring produce.

Breakfast Green Beans with Dill and Sumac

1 Heat the oil in a frying pan over a medium heat, add the spring onions and chilli and fry for 2–3 minutes to soften.

2 Add the asparagus and green beans and 2 tablespoons of water, cover and cook for 2–3 minutes until tender, then remove the lid and add the spinach. Re-cover and allow to wilt for a minute, then stir and season with salt and pepper.

3 Make 2 hollows in the vegetables and crack an egg into each one. Cover and cook for 2–3 minutes until the whites of the eggs have set and the yolk is still soft.

4 Remove from the heat, drizzle with the tahini and scatter with the dill and sumac. Serve with the yoghurt (if using) and flatbreads.

PREP 10 MINUTES/COOK 10 MINUTES

2 tbsp extra-virgin olive oil, plus extra for drizzling
60g spring onions (about 4), thinly sliced
1 red chilli, thinly sliced
160g asparagus spears, roughly chopped
160g green beans, roughly chopped
160g baby leaf spinach, roughly chopped
2 medium free-range eggs
1 tbsp tahini
10g fresh dill, chopped
pinch of sumac
sea salt and freshly ground black pepper

TO SERVE
4 tbsp natural yoghurt (optional)
2 flatbreads

The combination of smoky paprika with squash and red pepper is divine in this quick weekend favourite.

Fiery Frittata

1 Preheat the oven to 190°C/170°C fan/gas 5.

2 Heat the oil in a 20cm non-stick ovenproof frying pan over a low heat. Add the onion, squash and red pepper and fry very gently for 14–15 minutes until the squash is tender and the onions and peppers are softened.

3 Add the chilli and paprika and cook for a further 2–3 minutes.

4 Whisk the eggs and tomatoes in a bowl with salt and pepper. Stir into the pan and cook over a low heat for 2–3 minutes, agitating the egg with a spatula until it starts to set.

5 Transfer to the oven and cook for 8–10 minutes until fully set. Remove from the oven and serve with a scattering of coriander leaves.

PREP 15 MINUTES/COOK 25 MINUTES

75ml extra-virgin olive oil

160g red onion (about 1 medium), thinly sliced

200g deseeded, peeled butternut squash (about ¼), cut into 1cm cubes

180g deseeded red pepper (about 1 large), thinly sliced

1 red chilli, deseeded and thinly sliced

1 tsp smoked sweet paprika

5 medium free-range eggs

6 sun-dried tomatoes, finely chopped

sea salt and freshly ground black pepper

15g fresh coriander leaves, to serve

Cook's tip

Try blending the sun-dried tomatoes with the eggs in a bullet blender (or a regular blender) to give the frittata a lovely rich red colour.

I love a traditional shakshuka, but I also like to experiment with elements of the dish to make something unique and delicious, while amping up the vegetable content.

Spring Green and Broad Bean Shakshuka

1 Heat the oil in a frying pan over a low to medium heat, add the red onion and fry for 5 minutes until softened.

2 Add the garlic and cumin seeds and fry for a minute more, then add the passata, spring greens, oregano and 50ml water. Cover and cook for 2–3 minutes until the greens are just tender.

3 Add the peas and beans, re-cover and cook for 3–4 minutes more.

4 Season with salt and pepper and stir in most of the parsley. Make 2 hollows in the mixture and crack an egg into each. Cover and cook for 2–3 minutes until the whites of the eggs have set and the yolk is still soft.

5 Remove from the heat, scatter with the remaining parsley and serve with toasted pitta.

PREP 10 MINUTES/COOK 15–20 MINUTES

2 tbsp olive oil
100g red onion (about 1 small), thinly sliced
1 garlic clove, grated
1 tsp cumin seeds
200g passata
160g spring greens, shredded
leaves from 3 sprigs of oregano
160g fresh or frozen peas
160g fresh or frozen broad beans
25g fresh flat-leaf parsley, chopped
2 medium free-range eggs
sea salt and freshly ground black pepper
toasted pitta, to serve

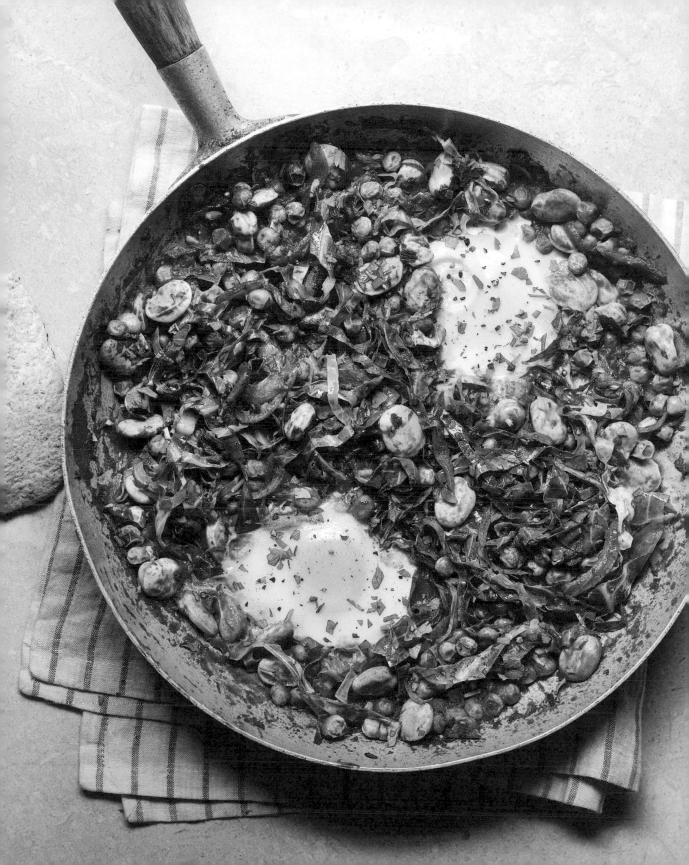

Za'atar is one of my favourite spice blends, and frittata is easily my favourite brunch dish. If you haven't tried combining the two, you're missing out.

Za'atar Frittata

1 Preheat the oven to 190°C/170°C fan/gas 5.

2 Heat the oil in a 20cm non-stick ovenproof frying pan over a low heat, add the potatoes and fry very gently for 8–10 minutes, turning them once, until golden and tender.

3 Add the leek to the pan and fry for 5 minutes until tender, then add the peas and spinach and allow the peas to defrost and the spinach to wilt for 2–3 minutes.

4 Whisk the eggs with the za'atar and salt and pepper. Add to the pan, mix, then cook over a low heat for 2–3 minutes, agitating the egg with a spatula until it starts to set.

5 Transfer to the oven and cook for 8–10 minutes until fully set. Remove from the oven and serve with the rocket and coriander.

PREP 10–15 MINUTES/COOK 25 MINUTES

75ml extra-virgin olive oil
300g new potatoes, sliced to the thickness of a pound coin
160g leeks (1 large or 2 small), thinly sliced
160g frozen peas
160g baby leaf spinach, finely chopped
5 medium free-range eggs
2 tsp za'atar
sea salt and freshly ground black pepper

TO SERVE
30g rocket leaves
15g fresh coriander leaves

Cook's tip
I blend the spinach with the eggs and za'atar in a bullet blender (or regular blender) before adding to the pan, for a vibrant green frittata.

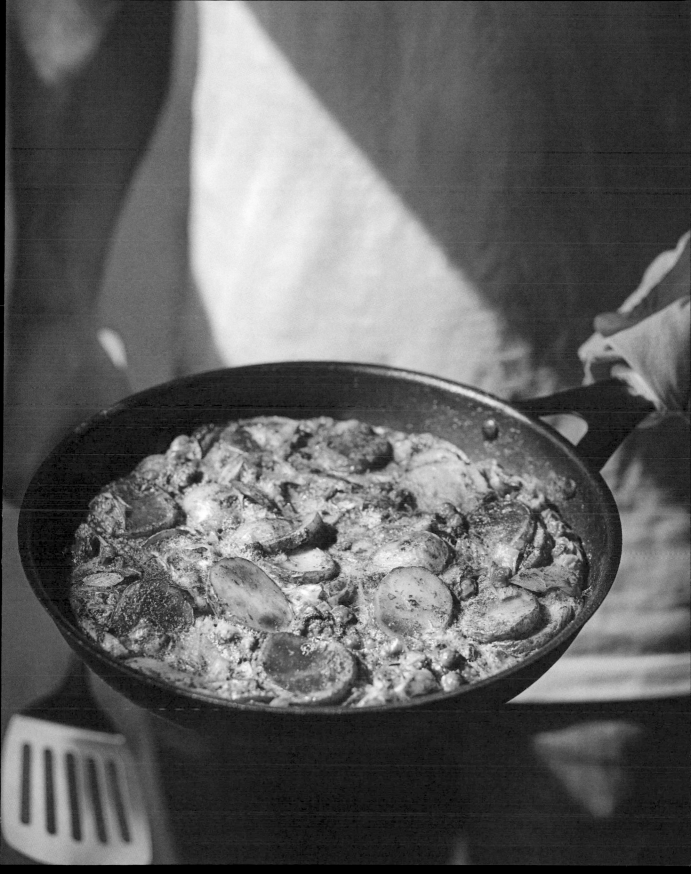

I sometimes swap veggie sausages for high-quality regular sausages in this dish, as they add even more flavour, but it's the quality of the sourdough that really makes this meal.

Sourdough and Veggie Sausage Bake

1 Preheat the oven to 200°C/180°C fan/gas 6.

2 Put the onions, leeks and rosemary leaves in a roasting tray, drizzle with the oil, season, and roast for 10 minutes until starting to soften.

3 Remove, nestle in the sausages and tomatoes and roast for another 15 minutes in the oven.

4 Turn the sausages, gently mix in the sourdough and drizzle over the stock. Return to the oven and roast for a further 15 minutes until the sausages are cooked and browned and the sourdough bread is sticky underneath and golden and crunchy on top.

5 Meanwhile, make the relish. Mix the parsley, capers and pine nuts with the chilli flakes (if using) and vinegar, then add the oil. Season and serve drizzled over the sausages.

PREP 20 MINUTES/COOK 40 MINUTES

160g red onion (about 1 medium), cut into wedges

200g leeks (2–3 small), thickly sliced on an angle

3 sprigs of rosemary, stripped

2 tbsp extra-virgin olive oil

4 veggie sausages

200g small vine tomatoes, halved

100g dark sourdough or rye bread, torn

2–3 tbsp vegetable stock (or water)

sea salt and freshly ground black pepper

FOR THE RELISH

25g fresh flat-leaf parsley, finely chopped

1 tbsp capers, drained, rinsed and finely chopped

1 tbsp toasted pine nuts, finely chopped

pinch of dried chilli flakes (optional)

2 tsp sherry vinegar

3 tbsp extra-virgin olive oil

Cook's tip

Make double the relish and mix half with natural yoghurt as a dip for chips or tortillas.

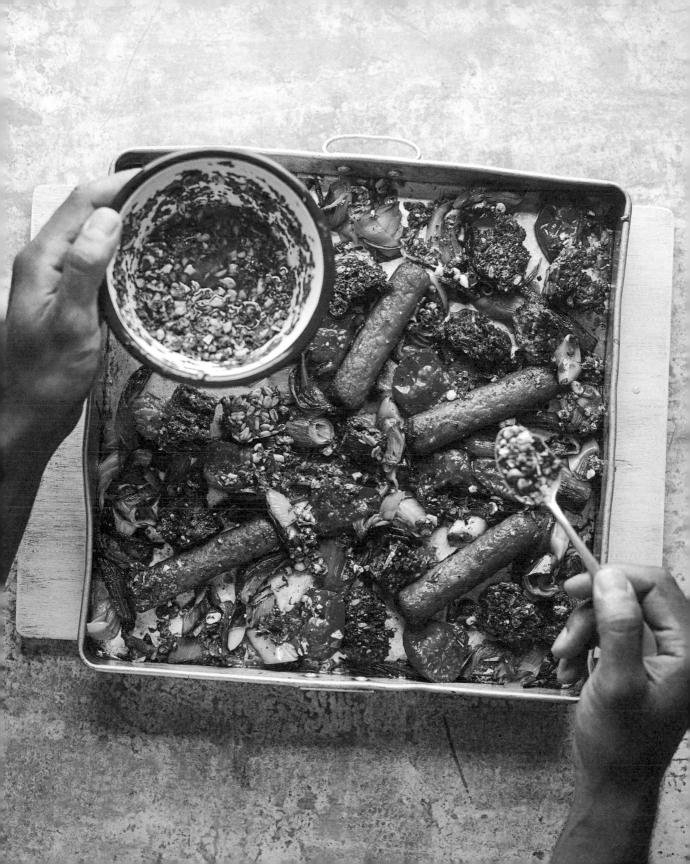

This one-pan Mexican-inspired dish, packed with gorgeous flavours from the cumin and hot paprika, will get your day off to a fiery start. And it's another recipe with four portions of veg per serving, too.

Huevos Rancheros

1 Heat the oil in a medium frying pan over a medium heat, add the onion and red pepper and fry gently for 10 minutes until softened.

2 Add the spices and fry for a minute more, then add the tomatoes, beans and 100ml water. Season with salt and pepper and cook for a further 10 minutes.

3 Make 2 hollows in the mixture and crack an egg into each. Cover and cook for 2–3 minutes until the whites are set and the yolks are still soft.

4 Remove from the heat and serve topped with the avocado and scattered with the coriander leaves, with warm tortillas for scooping.

PREP 10–15 MINUTES/COOK 25 MINUTES

2 tbsp extra-virgin olive oil
50g spring onions (about 3 or 4), thinly sliced
160g deseeded red pepper (about 1 large), sliced
1 tsp each hot and sweet smoked paprika
1 tsp cumin seeds
400g tin chopped tomatoes
400g tin black beans, drained and rinsed
2 medium free-range eggs
sea salt and freshly ground black pepper

TO SERVE
160g peeled and stoned avocado (1 large or 2 small), sliced
15g fresh coriander leaves, chopped
4 small corn tortillas, warmed in the oven or dry pan

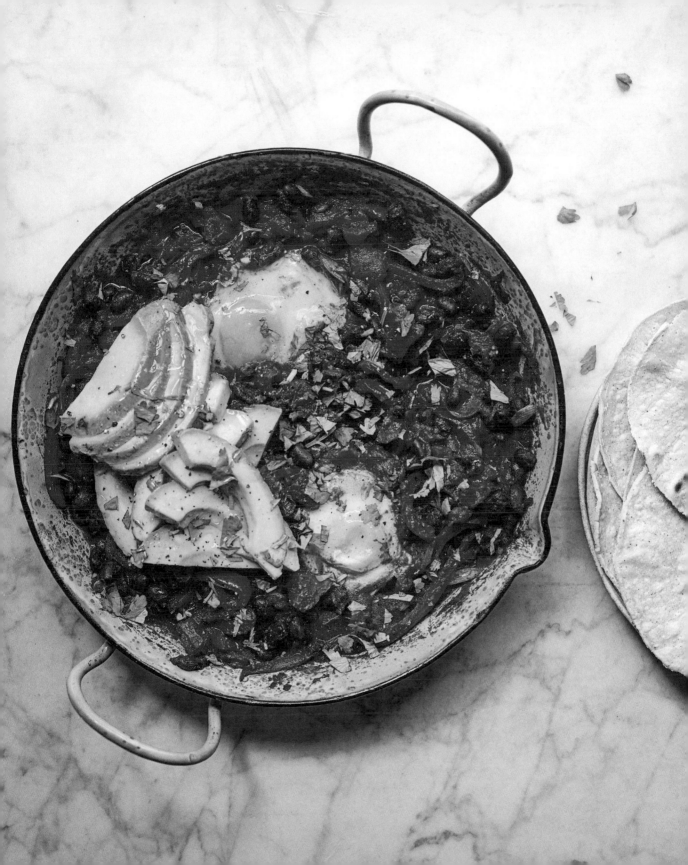

Fennel and nigella seeds accentuate the aromatic flavour of the vegetables in this dish. I love the ease of throwing it all into the tray, and experimenting with different dressing combinations.

Fennel and Mustard Potatoes

1 Preheat the oven to 200°C/180°C fan/gas 6.

2 Tip the potatoes, onion and fennel into a large roasting tray and drizzle with half the oil. Season with salt and pepper, add the spices and mix well, then roast in the oven for 20 minutes.

3 Add the cherry tomatoes and kale to the tray, drizzle with the remaining oil, toss to coat and roast for a further 15 minutes.

4 To make the dressing, whisk the mustard and vinegar together, season and add the oil and dill.

5 Once the vegetables are roasted and sticky, drizzle all over with half of the dressing. Make two hollows and crack the eggs into them. Return to the oven to bake for 5–6 minutes more, until the whites are set and the yolks are still soft but not runny. Serve with the rest of the dressing to drizzle over.

PREP 10–15 MINUTES/COOK 40 MINUTES

200g baby new potatoes, halved

160g red onion (about 1 medium), cut into wedges

200–250g fennel (about 1 bulb), cut into thin wedges

3 tbsp extra-virgin olive oil

1 tsp nigella seeds

1 tsp fennel seeds

200g cherry tomatoes, halved

80g trimmed kale, torn

2 medium free-range eggs

sea salt and freshly ground black pepper

FOR THE DRESSING

2 tsp Dijon mustard

1 tbsp white wine vinegar

3 tbsp extra-virgin olive oil

10g dill (or fronds from the fennel), finely chopped

I used to love kedgeree as a child, and still do. The wonderful curry spices in this dish are a welcome match for brown rice and they jazz up tons of green vegetables.

Spicy Salmon Kedgeree

1 Preheat the oven to 200°C/180°C fan/gas 6.

2 Put the oil, rice, spring onions, ginger and spices in a large, deep roasting tray (about 23cm across, 3cm deep). Add the stock and season with salt and pepper. Stir, cover tightly with foil and cook in the oven for 25 minutes.

3 After 25 minutes, reduce the oven temperature to 190°C/170°C fan/gas 5. Uncover, stir in the cavolo nero and peas, then top with the broccoli and salmon. Re-cover and return to the oven for 8–10 minutes, until the salmon is just cooked and the rice and veggies are tender.

4 Remove from the oven and serve scattered with the red chilli, coriander and flaked almonds.

PREP 15 MINUTES/COOK 35 MINUTES

2 tbsp extra-virgin olive oil
120g brown rice, rinsed
75g spring onions (about 5), thinly sliced
50g piece of root ginger (about 5cm), grated
2 tsp medium curry powder
pinch of dried chilli flakes
2 cardamom pods, bashed
1 vegetable stock cube dissolved in 400ml boiling water
160g trimmed cavolo nero, shredded
160g fresh or frozen peas
160g Tenderstem broccoli
200g skinless salmon fillets (about 2 small)
sea salt and freshly ground black pepper

TO SERVE
1 long red chilli, thinly sliced
15g fresh coriander leaves, torn
15g flaked almonds

Variation

You could use a tin of good-quality tuna fish in olive oil, flaked, instead of salmon.

Ever since my trip to Mexico during medical school I've always loved the fresh flavours of the cuisine and use of citrus to cut through hearty meals. This is a dish I have for breakfast but it works easily for dinner too!

Breakfast Burritos

1 Preheat the oven to 220°C/200°C fan/gas 7.

2 Mix the oil, rice, spring onions, coriander stalks, spices and beans in a roasting tray. Crumble in the stock cube, season with salt and pepper, pour in the boiling water and stir. Cover tightly with foil and cook in the oven for 30 minutes.

3 Add the sweetcorn, stir, re-cover and return to the oven for about 10 minutes, remove from the heat and rest, covered, for 5 minutes. Fold in the coriander leaves.

4 Meanwhile, roughly mash the avocado and mix in the tomatoes, lemon juice and some seasoning.

5 Spoon the rice and beans onto warmed tortillas and top with the guacamole and sour cream (if using). Fold into burritos and serve.

Cook's tip
You can cook this in an ovenproof pan with a lid if you wanted to save on foil.

PREP 10 MINUTES/COOK 45 MINUTES

1 tbsp extra-virgin olive oil
100g brown rice, rinsed
75g spring onions (about 5), finely chopped
25g fresh coriander, leaves and stalks chopped
1 tsp ground cumin
1 tsp hot smoked paprika
400g tin kidney beans, drained and rinsed
1 vegetable stock cube
375ml boiling water
160g sweetcorn kernels (fresh or frozen)
sea salt and freshly ground black pepper

FOR THE GUACAMOLE
160g peeled and stoned avocado (1 large or 2 small)
50g cherry tomatoes, finely chopped
squeeze of lemon juice

TO SERVE
4 wholemeal tortillas, warmed
4 tbsp sour cream (optional)

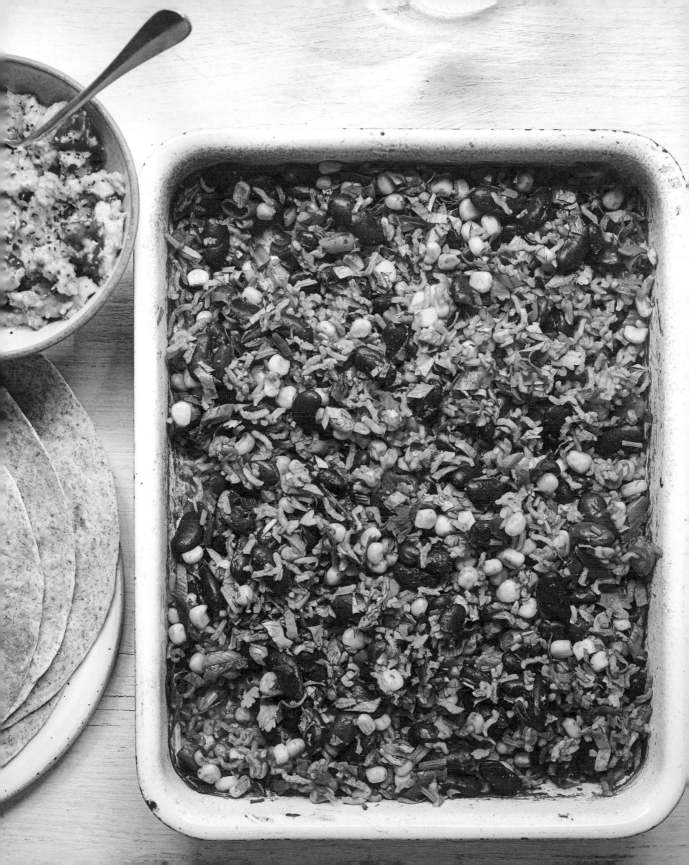

Salads

This classic chicken salad makes a perfect summer lunch, but also works well as a light dinner. The bitter red radicchio leaves are mellowed with the aromatic spice of star anise and the luxurious creamy tahini dressing.

Ginger Chicken Salad with Tahini Ranch Dressing

1 Put the ginger, lemongrass and star anise in a pan of boiling water. Add the chicken (ensuring there is enough water to cover the chicken) bring to a simmer and cook for 15 minutes until the chicken is just cooked.

2 Remove the chicken from the cooking water, set aside and allow to rest. Reserve 75ml of the cooking water.

3 To make the dressing, whisk the tahini with the garlic, lemon juice and reserved cooking water. Gradually whisk in the oil then season with salt and pepper and stir in the dill.

4 Arrange the salad leaves and radishes on a platter. Tear the poached chicken into strips and place on top of the leaves. Drizzle with the dressing and scatter with the sesame seeds.

PREP 15 MINUTES/COOK 20 MINUTES

60g piece of root ginger (about 6cm), roughly chopped
1 stick of lemongrass, bruised
1 star anise
150g skinless chicken breast
160g radicchio leaves
50g watercress
160g radishes, thinly sliced or quartered
1 tbsp sesame seeds
sea salt and freshly ground black pepper

FOR THE TAHINI RANCH DRESSING
60g tahini
1 garlic clove, grated
juice of ½ lemon
2 tbsp extra-virgin olive oil
1 tbsp finely chopped dill

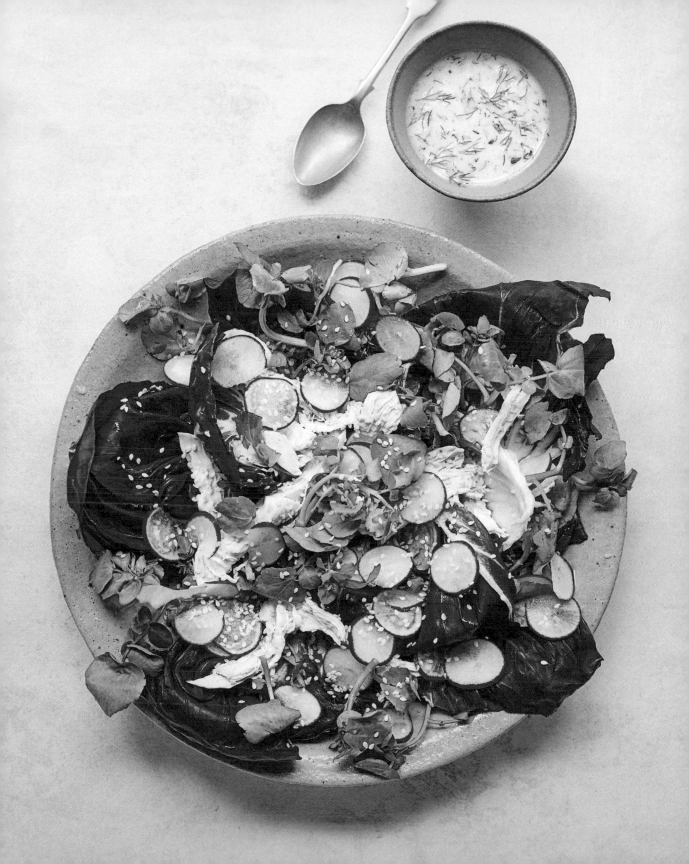

The combination of sumac and paprika – a beautiful blend of heat and citrus flavour – really brings this simple dish to life!

Mixed Herb Salad with Paprika and Sumac

1 Spoon the hummus onto two plates. Toss the watercress, lettuce, herbs and beans together and arrange on top of the hummus.

2 Toast the pumpkin seeds in a dry frying pan for a couple of minutes until golden.

3 Take off the heat, add the spices, season well with salt and pepper and toss together.

4 Squeeze the lemon juice over the salad, sprinkle over the toasted seeds and spices and drizzle with the extra-virgin olive oil.

Cook's tip

Toss the gem lettuce leaves in a little lemon juice or white wine vinegar before placing them on the hummus, for extra tang.

PREP 10 MINUTES/COOK 2 MINUTES

100g hummus

160g watercress

160g baby gem lettuce (about 1 head), leaves separated

20g mixed fresh soft herbs (parsley, dill, coriander, tarragon), torn

400g tin white beans, drained and rinsed

60g pumpkin seeds

½ tsp smoked paprika

1 tsp sumac

½ lemon

1 tbsp extra-virgin olive oil

sea salt and freshly ground black pepper

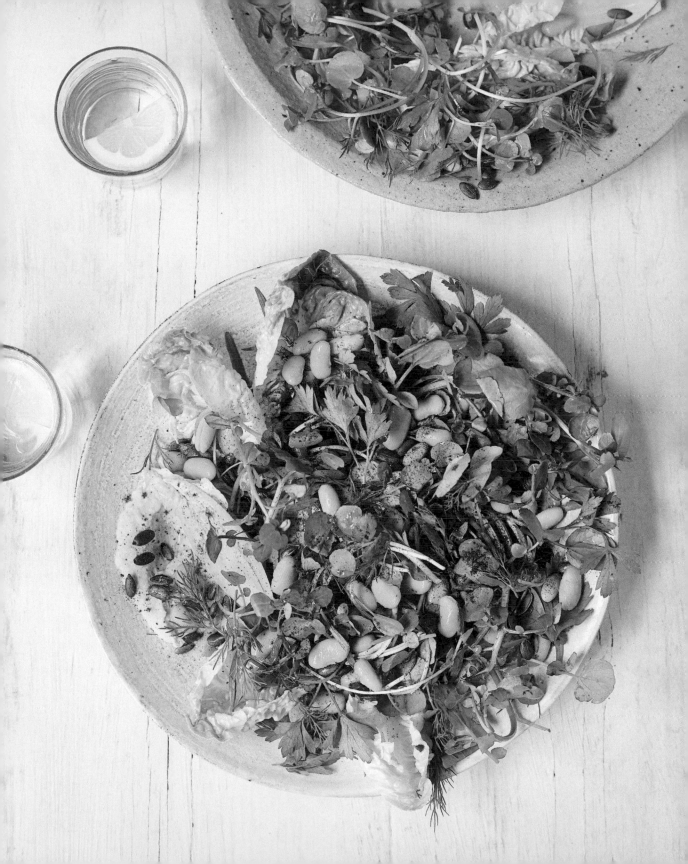

This delicate, luxurious salad uses a fantastic flavour combination of allspice, coriander seed and bittersweet pomegranate molasses to make a star dish that takes almost no mental effort to pull together.

Roasted Carrot Salad with Allspice, Cinnamon and Pistachio

1 Preheat the oven to 180°C/160°C fan/gas 4.

2 Toss the carrots in the oil and the spices in a roasting tray, season with salt and pepper and roast in the oven for 35 minutes until tender.

3 Toss the lentils, pistachios, watercress and pomegranate molasses into the roasted carrots. Serve scattered with the feta and mint and a drizzle more oil.

Variation

Use ¼ teaspoon ground allspice instead of the berries if you don't have them.

PREP 10 MINUTES/COOK 35 MINUTES

250g carrots (2–3 small), cut into batons

1 tbsp extra-virgin olive oil, plus extra for drizzling

5 allspice berries, roughly crushed

¼ tsp ground cinnamon

1 tsp coriander seeds, roughly crushed

160g cooked puy lentils (from a tin or packet)

60g shelled, unsalted pistachios, roughly chopped

160g watercress, torn

2 tsp pomegranate molasses

sea salt and freshly ground black pepper

TO SERVE

75g feta cheese, crumbled

15g fresh mint leaves, chopped

Preserved lemon can now be found in most supermarkets. It has a beautiful perfume of fresh lemonade that pairs perfectly with fresh green leaves and broad beans. You could also serve this with some plain bulghur wheat or couscous.

Green Leaves and Broad Beans with Preserved Lemon and Paprika

1 Bring a saucepan of water to the boil and blanch the broad beans for 2–3 minutes. Drain and refresh under cold running water.

2 Tip the beans into a bowl and toss with the spinach, parsley and preserved lemon.

3 Whisk the vinegar with the paprika and some salt and pepper. Whisk in the oil, then pour over the salad and toss together. Scatter over the nuts and serve.

PREP 5 MINUTES/COOK 3 MINUTES

160g broad beans (fresh or frozen)
160g baby spinach leaves, roughly chopped
20g fresh flat-leaf parsley leaves
40g preserved lemon rind, finely chopped
1 tbsp balsamic vinegar
½ tsp smoked paprika
2 tbsp extra-virgin olive oil
60g walnuts, roughly chopped
sea salt and freshly ground black pepper

Cook's tips

Dry-toast the walnuts for an added smoky flavour. If you have time, double-pod the broad beans after blanching and running under cold water to reveal the bright green bean inside.

I love this technique for making a warm dressing. Sizzling the garlic in the hot oil with the spices builds a beautiful aroma, and the umami flavour of the anchovy is divine.

Butter Bean Salad with Fried Garlic and Hazelnut Dressing

1 Heat the olive oil in a small pan over a low heat. Add the chopped hazelnuts and anchovy fillets and cook gently for 3–4 minutes until the anchovies dissolve and the nuts have coloured.

2 Remove from the heat and add the nigella seeds, cumin seeds and chilli flakes, then grate the garlic straight into the hot oil. Stir, allowing the garlic to cook gently in the residual heat for about 1 minute.

3 Add the butter beans to the same pan and stir to warm a little.

4 Toss the leaves and the warm beans in a salad bowl and add a squeeze of lemon juice before serving.

PREP 10 MINUTES/COOK 3–4 MINUTES

50ml extra-virgin olive oil
60g hazelnuts, roughly chopped
3 anchovy fillets in oil, from a jar
1 tsp nigella seeds
1 tsp cumin seeds
pinch of dried chilli flakes
1 garlic clove, peeled
400g tin butter beans, drained and rinsed
80g rocket leaves, roughly chopped
80g pea shoot leaves, roughly chopped
juice of ½ lemon

Variation

To make this completely plant-based, try using 2 teaspoons of white miso paste instead of the anchovy fillets.

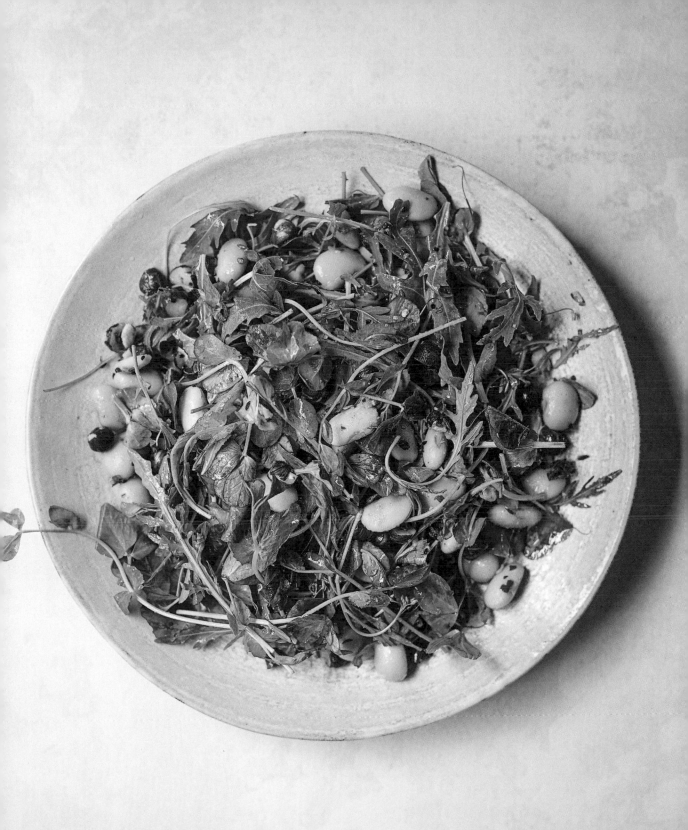

I love this delicious crumb on the delicate fish. You can also try it with a Cajun spice blend or garam masala.

Herb and Walnut Crumbed Fish with Pickled Red Cabbage

1 Preheat the oven to 200°C/180°C fan/gas 6.

2 Put the cabbage in a large bowl. Mix the vinegar with the fennel seeds and honey or sugar and season. Add the boiling water, pour the mixture over the cabbage and toss to combine. Set aside for 30 minutes.

3 Finely chop most of the walnuts with the dried herbs, chilli flakes and breadcrumbs and season.

4 Put the fish on a baking tray and press the crumb over the top to coat, drizzle with the oil and bake in the oven for 10–12 minutes, until the crumb is golden and the fish is just cooked and opaque.

5 Set the peas and lettuce on two plates, top with the cabbage and fish. Scatter with the remaining walnuts and drizzle with oil.

PREP 15 MINUTES, PLUS 30 MINUTES PICKLING/COOK 10–12 MINUTES

60g walnut pieces
½ tsp dried oregano
½ tsp dried thyme
½ tsp dried chilli flakes
40g fine wholemeal breadcrumbs
2 x 175g skinless white fish fillets (such as cod or haddock)
4 tbsp extra-virgin olive oil, plus extra for drizzling
160g frozen peas, defrosted
50g lamb's lettuce
sea salt and freshly ground black pepper

FOR THE PICKLED RED CABBAGE
160g red cabbage (about ¼), very thinly sliced
3 tbsp white wine vinegar
1 tsp fennel seeds
1 tbsp honey or sugar
50ml boiling water

Cook's tip
You can use red cabbage sauerkraut instead of pickling your own cabbage to save time.

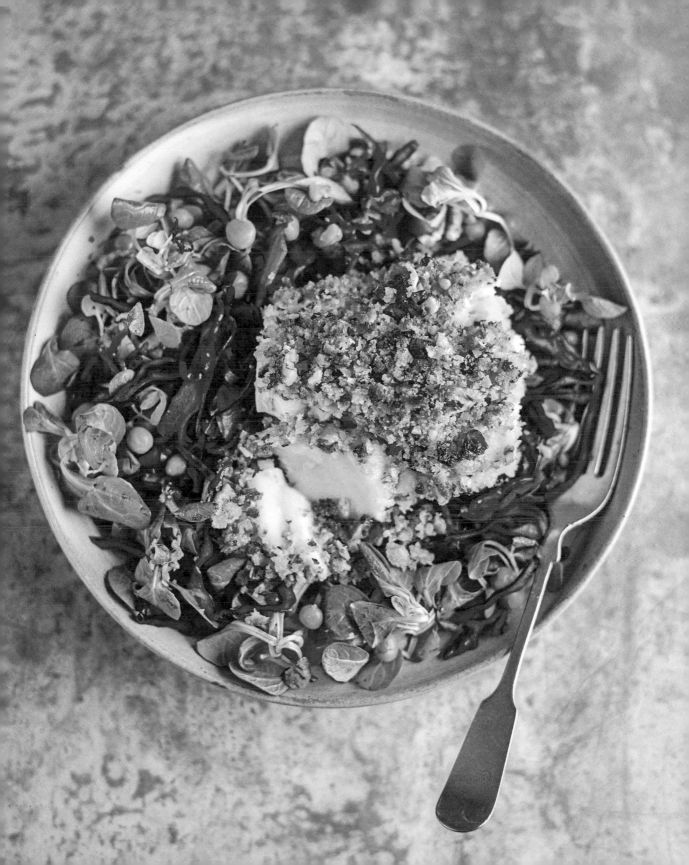

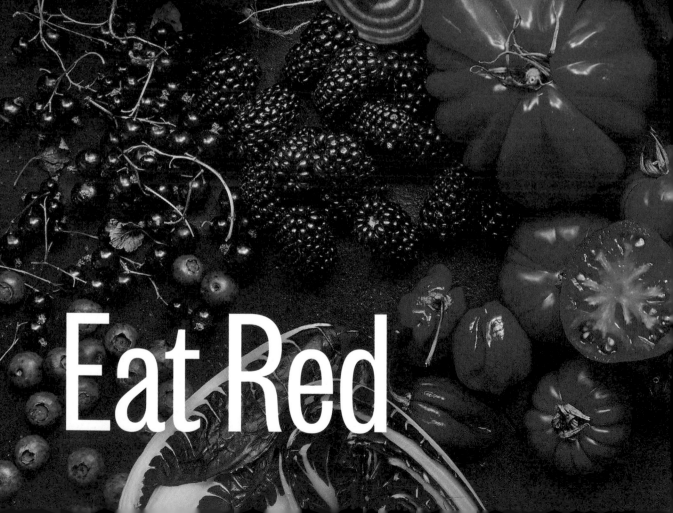

Eat Red

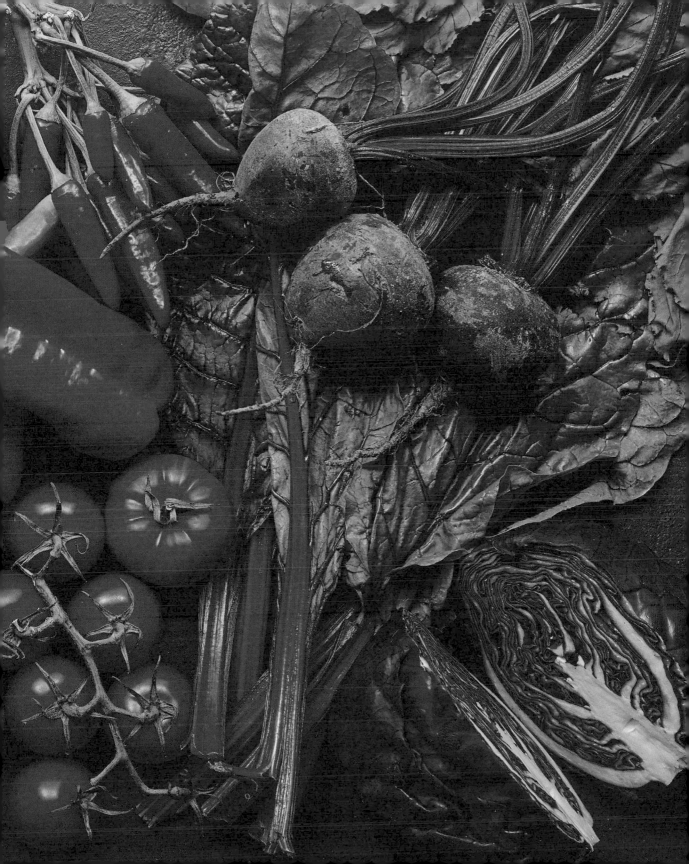

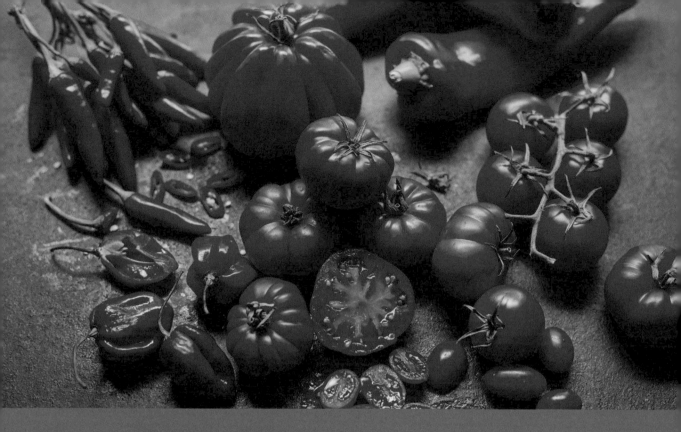

Red foods feature a wide spectrum of fruit and vegetables including beetroot, berries, chard, onion, carrot, purple broccoli and cabbage. The red colours represent a multitude of plant chemical categories that include the betalains and anthocyanins that have been shown to relax blood vessels and contribute to improving blood pressure in both lab studies and human trials.

Of particular interest to me are berries, including blackberries, blueberries and blackcurrants. These ingredients are particularly rich sources of polyphenols, including resveratrol and quercetin that are well known to have anti-inflammatory properties, but also have a role in the production of neurotrophic factors that help support the growth of brain cells that may help prevent dementia and improve cognition.

These studies are based on population observations that demonstrate the lower incidence of brain disease in those who eat fruit and vegetables plentifully, so they are not the most robust. However, taking them together with other studies that examine how these plant chemicals exhibit their effects on the body, we begin to build a picture of how fruits and vegetables can improve sugar balance, enhance blood flow to the brain and potentially help with depression and reduce the risk of neurodegenerative conditions like dementia.

Berries may also have a positive effect on cells of the immune system: a number of studies have demonstrated that eating berries is associated with increased numbers of specialised immune cells involved in the initial response to infections and removing damaged mutated cells, an action that could help protect against cancer.

Peppers and chillies feature commonly in my recipes and they contain an abundance of phytonutrients including carotenoids, flavonoids, luteolin and mycertin as well as alkaloids called capsaicinoids that give them their heat. Chillies have been found to lessen pain perception in arthritis but the combination of chemicals in peppers may also have benefits for blood flow, which prevents high blood pressure.

I'm constantly adding tomatoes to my dishes, both cooked and fresh, to boost the nutrient profile of meals I make. Known for their lycopene content, a novel antioxidant that is actually better absorbed when tomatoes are cooked for longer, they are potent protectors of DNA damage and may even have the ability to prevent photo-damage from sunlight exposure (although minimising excessive exposure and using sun cream is still recommended). These chemicals in tomatoes, also found in watermelon and guava, have been shown to arrest cancer cell growth. There is heightened interest specifically for their effects on slow-growing prostate cancers (although it's hard to determine the direct effects on cancer considering the minimal research available).

It's important to remember that foods are not the sum of individual plant chemicals, micronutrients and macronutrients we can measure, but rather the complex arrangement and combination of all these nutrients, perfected by nature, that collectively enhance our health. These foods are digested in the mouth and stomach by different enzymes, which create new chemicals from the collection of anthocyanins, flavonoids and flavanols found in the original food. Again, these are metabolised further in the gut by microbes to reveal completely novel chemicals far removed from the original polyphenols we started with.

Thousands of different types of plant chemicals exist, and only a small collection of them have been studied in detail, which is why it's important to maintain perspective of how complicated nutritional science is and why it's the basic message of eating more colour that matters. It's also near impossible to demonstrate what aspect of food is responsible for the associations we see with greater fruit and vegetable consumption and improved heart, brain and mental health when these ingredients are such complex, intricate structures.

We eat with our eyes, and I love the stunning beauty of this salad. It shouts 'healthy', yet is so delicious and satisfying.

The Red One

1 Preheat the oven to 200°C/180°C fan/gas 6.

2 Toss the beetroot in a roasting tray with half of the oil, the cumin, nigella and pumpkin seeds and plenty of salt and pepper.

3 Roast in the oven for 20 minutes, then turn the beetroot, add the sourdough to the tray and drizzle with the remaining tablespoon of oil. Roast for a further 10–15 minutes until the beetroot is tender and the bread golden and crisp.

4 Remove from the oven and leave to cool in the tray.

5 Once cooled, tip into a bowl and muddle through the radicchio, tomatoes and tarragon. Drizzle with a little more oil and serve.

Variation

Try roasting other vegetables such as pumpkin, parsnip or fennel, instead of the beetroot.

PREP 10 MINUTES/COOK 35 MINUTES

200g beetroot (3–4 small), cut into wedges
2 tbsp extra-virgin olive oil, plus extra for drizzling
1 tsp cumin seeds
1 tsp nigella seeds
40g pumpkin seeds
100g sourdough bread, torn
160g radicchio, roughly chopped
200g small or cherry vine tomatoes, halved or quartered
15g fresh tarragon leaves
sea salt and freshly ground black pepper

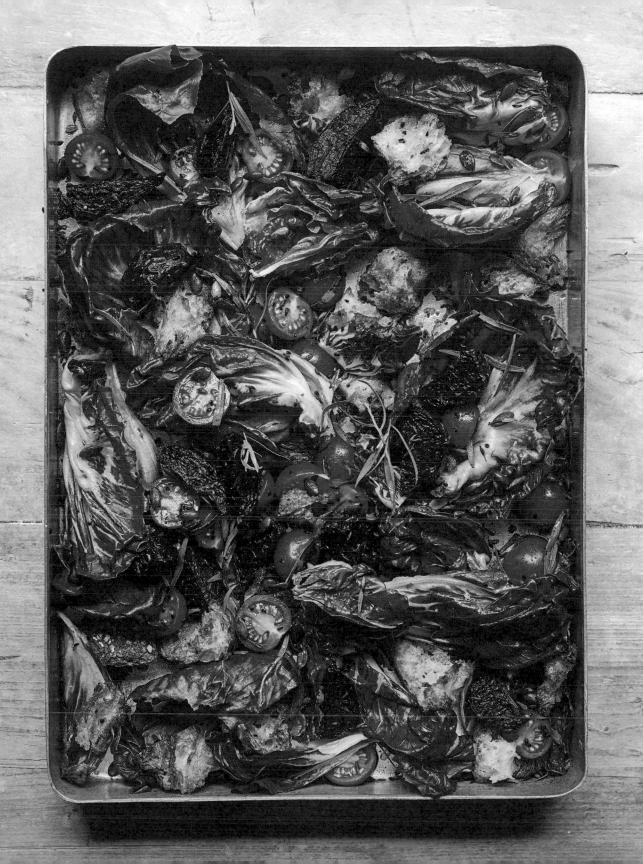

This satisfying Southern-style dish is simple to whip up and uses a beautiful mix of green aromatic herbs that work really well with the hint of spice delivered by the chilli flakes.

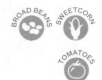

Southern-style Succotash Salad

1 Heat the oil in a sauté pan or shallow casserole dish over a medium heat, add the celery and garlic and fry for 2–3 minutes until coloured.

2 Add the beans and the corn, season well with salt and pepper and cook for 3–5 minutes until the corn is golden. Add the butter and stir through, then take off the heat and add the tomatoes.

3 Arrange the lamb's lettuce or other leaves over a serving plate, top with the succotash, scatter with the herbs and chili flakes and serve.

Cook's tip

Try topping this with corn nuts or fried fava (broad) beans for extra crunch.

Variation

Swap tinned broad beans for tinned butter beans if you like.

PREP 5–10 MINUTES / COOK 10 MINUTES

2 tbsp extra-virgin olive oil
50g celery (about 1 stalk), diced
2 garlic cloves, grated
400g tin broad beans, drained and rinsed
160g sweetcorn kernels (either sliced from a cob or frozen)
2 tsp unsalted butter
160g cherry tomatoes, sliced in half
50g lamb's lettuce or other small leaves
sea salt and freshly ground black pepper

TO SERVE
15g fresh tarragon leaves, torn
15g fresh basil leaves, torn
pinch of dried chilli flakes

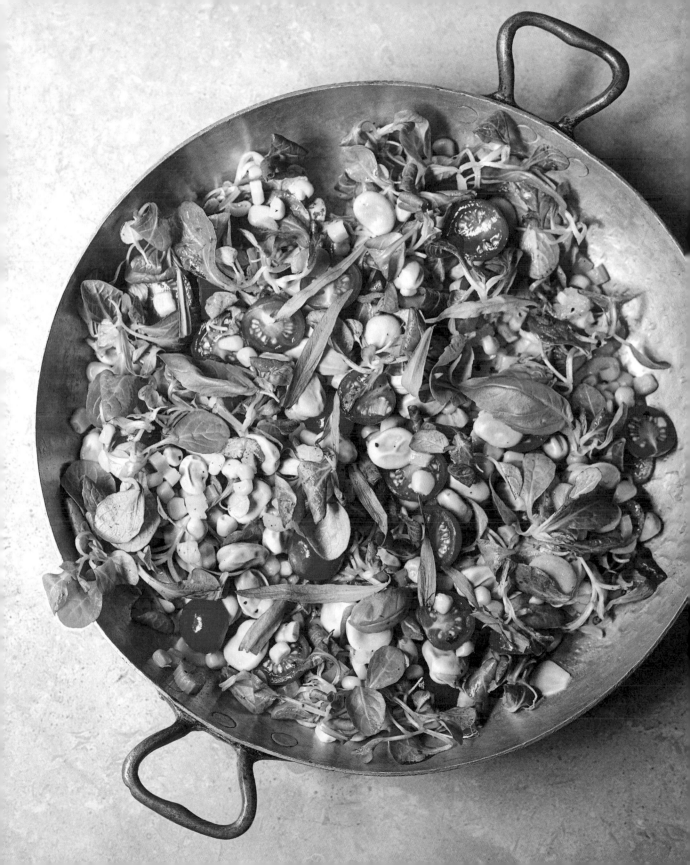

Pomegranate molasses and harissa are a perfect match for a salad that delivers effortless flavour.

Harissa Green Bean Salad

1 Preheat the oven to 200°C/180°C fan/gas 6.

2 Toss the beans and nuts in a roasting tray with the garlic, cumin seeds, harissa and olive oil. Season well with salt and pepper and roast in the oven for 20 minutes.

3 Remove from the oven, add the spinach and parsley to the tray and stir to wilt.

4 Drizzle with the pomegranate molasses and scatter with pomegranate seeds to serve.

PREP 5 MINUTES/COOK 20 MINUTES

200g green beans
60g hazelnuts, roughly chopped
2 garlic cloves, bashed or chopped
1 tsp cumin seeds
1 tbsp rose harissa paste (or regular harissa)
2 tbsp extra-virgin olive oil
160g baby leaf spinach, roughly chopped
20g fresh flat-leaf parsley, roughly chopped
2 tsp pomegranate molasses
50g pomegranate seeds
sea salt and freshly ground black pepper

Cook's tip

This would be delicious served with griddled halloumi or crumbled feta cheese.

The salty-sweet combination of capers with chopped pecans is a fantastic match for the bitter chicory. The union of these ingredients creates a delicious flavour base that really makes the dish sing.

Grilled Chicory Salad with Fennel, Capers and Pecans

1 Heat a griddle pan over a high heat. Brush or rub the chicory wedges with olive oil and sear on the griddle on both sides for 2–3 minutes until charred. Roughly chop and tip into a bowl.

2 Toss with the fennel, lentils, nuts, capers and lemon segments.

3 Whisk the lemon juice with plenty of salt and pepper, the pinch of sugar and the rest of the olive oil and pour over the salad.

4 Toss together and scatter with the dill or reserved fennel fronds.

PREP 10 MINUTES/COOK 5 MINUTES

160g red chicory, quartered
2 tbsp extra-virgin olive oil
160g fennel (about 1 small bulb), finely shaved or sliced
160g cooked puy lentils (from a tin or packet)
40g pecans, roughly chopped
20g capers, drained and rinsed
1 lemon, segmented (juice reserved)
a pinch of sugar or 1 tsp honey
1 tbsp chopped fresh dill or reserved fennel fronds
sea salt and freshly ground black pepper

The spicy kimchi dressing blended with sweet grated apple and carrot creates a beautiful fiery and crunchy salad.

Kimchi Slaw with Greens and Sriracha Mayo

1 Tip the kimchi into a sieve over a bowl, lightly squeeze out the juice and set aside. Tip the drained kimchi into a salad bowl.

2 Whisk the kimchi juice with the sesame oil, soy sauce, sriracha and mayonnaise and season to taste if it needs it.

3 To the salad bowl with the kimchi add the carrots, cabbage, apple and beansprouts, then pour over the dressing, reserving some, and mix well.

4 Garnish with coriander leaves and peanuts, and serve with a little extra drizzle of dressing.

PREP TIME 20 MINUTES

160g shop-bought kimchi
2 tsp sesame oil
1 tbsp soy sauce
1 tbsp sriracha
3 tbsp mayonnaise
160g carrots (1 large or 2 small), julienned or coarsely grated
160g pointed cabbage (about ½ head), finely shredded
120g apple (about 1 small), julienned or coarsely grated
50g beansprouts
sea salt (optional)

TO SERVE
15g fresh coriander leaves, roughly chopped
30g unsalted roasted peanuts, chopped

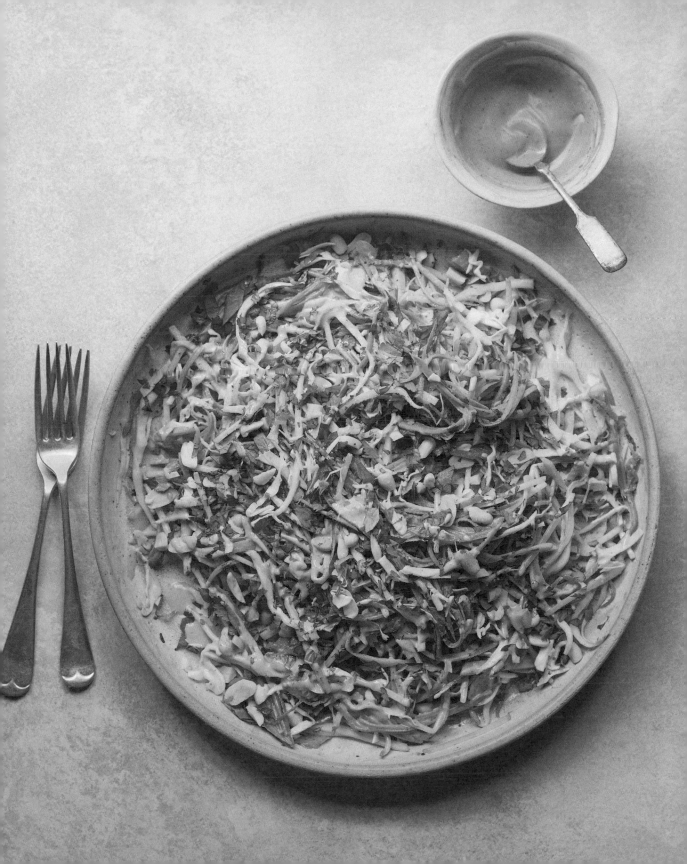

This is my go-to, super-simple midweek salad, when I want something light, flavourful and packed full of nutrients.

Mixed Bean Salad with a Spicy Tarragon and Oregano Dressing

1 Bring a saucepan of water to the boil, add the runner beans and sugar snap peas and blanch for 3–4 minutes until just tender. Drain and refresh under cold running water until just a little warm, then dry well and tip into a bowl.

2 Add the rest of the ingredients, mix well with your hands, season with salt and pepper, then serve.

Variation

This would also work with a Herbes de Provence mix instead of the dried oregano, or 2 teaspoons of fresh, sliced oregano leaves.

PREP 5 MINUTES/COOK 5 MINUTES

160g runner beans, sliced on the angle
160g sugar snap peas
400g tin mixed beans, drained and rinsed
½ tsp dried oregano
10g fresh tarragon leaves, chopped
3 tbsp extra-virgin olive oil
60g pitted Kalamata olives, halved
finely grated zest and juice of ½ lemon
good pinch of dried chilli flakes
sea salt and freshly ground black pepper

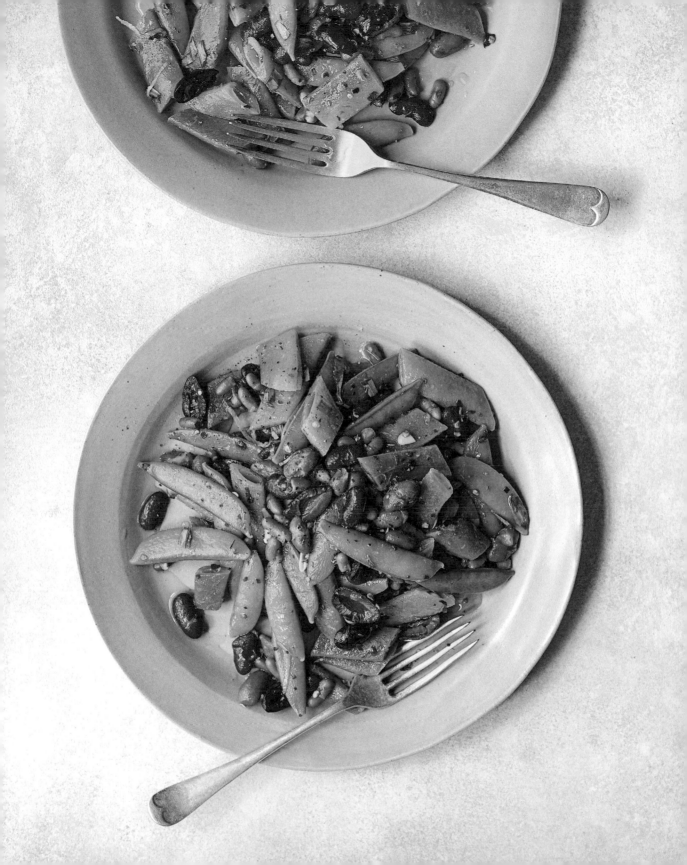

Whole
Grains

I remember cooking this for the first time and thinking how unbelievably easy it was. Everything is prepped in the pan, there is minimal chopping and the nutritional value is brilliant. This will become your go-to dish!

Masala Rice with Sardines

1 Preheat the oven to 210°C/190°C fan/gas 7.

2 Put the rice, lentils, peas and spinach in a medium, shallow casserole dish. Pour over the boiling water, season with salt and pepper and stir in the spices. Top with the sardines, cover with a tight-fitting lid or foil and cook in the oven for 40 minutes.

3 Remove from the oven and leave to stand, covered, for 5 minutes, then garnish with the chilli and coriander and serve with lime wedges to squeeze over.

PREP 10 MINUTES / COOK 40 MINUTES

100g brown basmati rice, rinsed
160g dried green speckled lentils, rinsed
160g frozen peas
160g spinach
600ml boiling water
1 tbsp garam masala
1 tsp ground turmeric
½ tsp dried chilli flakes
120g tin sardines (in oil or water), drained
sea salt and freshly ground black pepper

TO SERVE
1 red chilli, finely chopped
15g fresh coriander leaves, torn
1 lime, cut into wedges

Variation

Try this with harissa paste instead of garam masala for an easy Middle Eastern twist.

This autumnal dish is a perfect way to use seasonal root vegetables like swede and parsnip. I always keep dried mushrooms to hand, as they are an easy way to add depth of flavour to hearty dishes like this.

Wild Mushroom Barley and Beans

1 Put the mushrooms in a heatproof bowl, pour over 300ml of the boiling water and leave for 10 minutes.

2 While the mushrooms soak, heat the oil in a lidded sauté pan or casserole over a medium heat, add the pearl barley and root veg and cook for 3–4 minutes.

3 Drain the mushrooms, reserving the liquid, and roughly chop. Add the sun-dried tomatoes, parsley stalks and mushrooms to the pan.

4 Crumble the stock cube into the pan and add the remaining 200ml boiling water with the mushroom soaking liquid (discard the grit).

5 Season, cover and simmer for 30 minutes until most of the stock has been absorbed (you may need to add a little more boiling water).

6 Stir in the beans to warm through, remove from the heat and serve with the rocket and parsley leaves.

PREP 15 MINUTES/COOK 35 MINUTES

40g dried mixed wild mushrooms
500ml boiling water
2 tbsp olive oil
80g pearl barley
160g carrots (1 large or 2 small), cut into 1cm pieces
160g swede or parsnip, cut into 1cm pieces
50g sun-dried tomatoes, roughly chopped
20g fresh flat-leaf parsley, stalks and leaves chopped
½ vegetable stock cube
400g tin haricot beans, drained and rinsed
sea salt and freshly ground black pepper
50g wild rocket leaves, to serve

Jewelled rice, the epitome of luxurious home cooking, combining saffron, barberries and nuts, was a favourite in my household when I was growing up. This version of the original is far quicker and it does not disappoint!

Fragrant Jewelled Rice

1 Put a lidded casserole dish over a medium heat and add 1 tablespoon of the olive oil, the rice, spices, chickpeas, carrots and spring onions and stir for 1 minute to allow the flavours to mingle.

2 Add the orange zest and juice, crumble in the stock cube, add plenty of salt and pepper and pour over the boiling water. Stir, cover and simmer for 35 minutes.

3 Remove from the heat, fold in the courgettes, cherries or barberries, nuts, parsley and the remaining extra-virgin olive oil and serve.

Cook's tip

Scatter a generous pinch of dried rose petals over the finished dish to add floral fragrance and flavour.

PREP 10 MINUTES/COOK 35 MINUTES

2 tbsp extra-virgin olive oil

100g brown basmati rice, rinsed

1 cinnamon stick

3 cardamom pods, crushed

½ tsp ground turmeric

a few saffron strands (optional)

400g tin chickpeas, drained and rinsed

160g carrots (1 large or 2 small), julienned or coarsely grated

75g spring onions (about 5), finely chopped, plus extra to garnish

finely grated zest and juice of 1 orange

1 vegetable stock cube

450ml boiling water

160g courgettes (2 medium), julienned or peeled into thin ribbons

20g sour cherries or barberries

20g flaked almonds

20g shelled, unsalted pistachios, roughly chopped

15g fresh flat-leaf parsley, chopped

sea salt and freshly ground black pepper

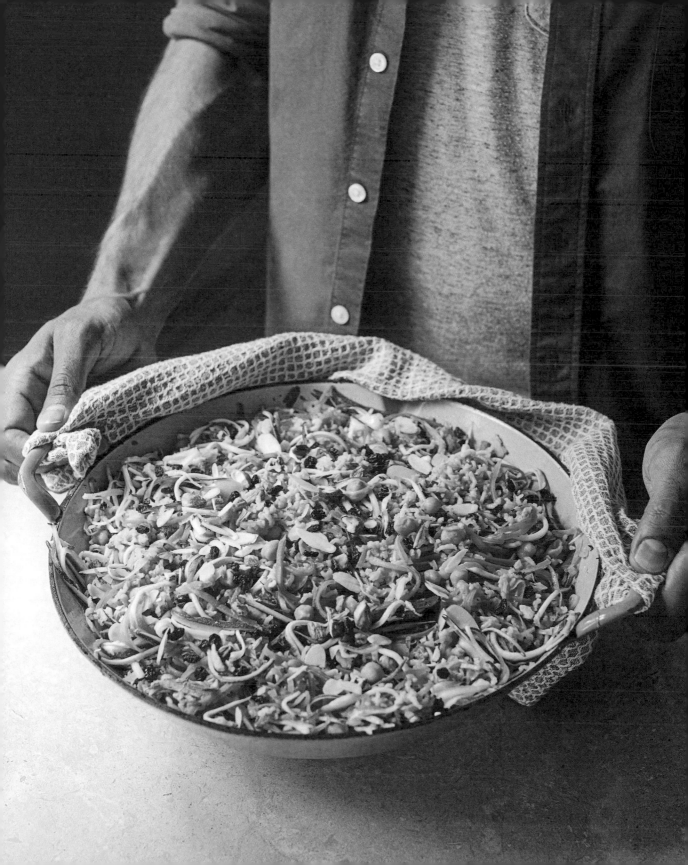

Another takeaway favourite of mine. This method of cooking wholegrains in the oven is such a doddle – it allows the flavours to really intensify, and builds incredible aromas in your kitchen.

Nasi Goreng

1 Preheat the oven to 210°C/190°C fan/gas 7.

2 In a lidded casserole dish, mix the rice with the nasi goreng paste, add the lemongrass, ginger, soy sauce, red pepper and carrots. Pour over the boiling water, season with salt and pepper and stir. Cover and bake in the oven for 35 minutes.

3 Remove from the oven, leave to stand (covered) for 5 minutes, then fold in the beansprouts.

4 Serve with the chilli, coriander and peanuts scattered over, with lime wedges for squeezing.

Cook's tip

If nasi goreng paste is hard to find, you can use a different spice blends such as a laksa or chilli bean paste instead.

PREP 10–15 MINUTES/COOK 35 MINUTES

100g brown rice, rinsed

3 tbsp nasi goreng spice paste

1 stick of lemongrass, bashed with a rolling pin

25g piece of root ginger (about 2.5cm), grated

1 tbsp soy sauce

160g deseeded red pepper (about 1 large), thinly sliced

160g carrots (1 large or 2 small), shredded or coarsely grated

350ml boiling water

160g beansprouts

sea salt and freshly ground black pepper

TO SERVE

1 long red chilli, thinly sliced

20g fresh coriander leaves, chopped

20g unsalted peanuts, roughly chopped

1 lime, cut into wedges

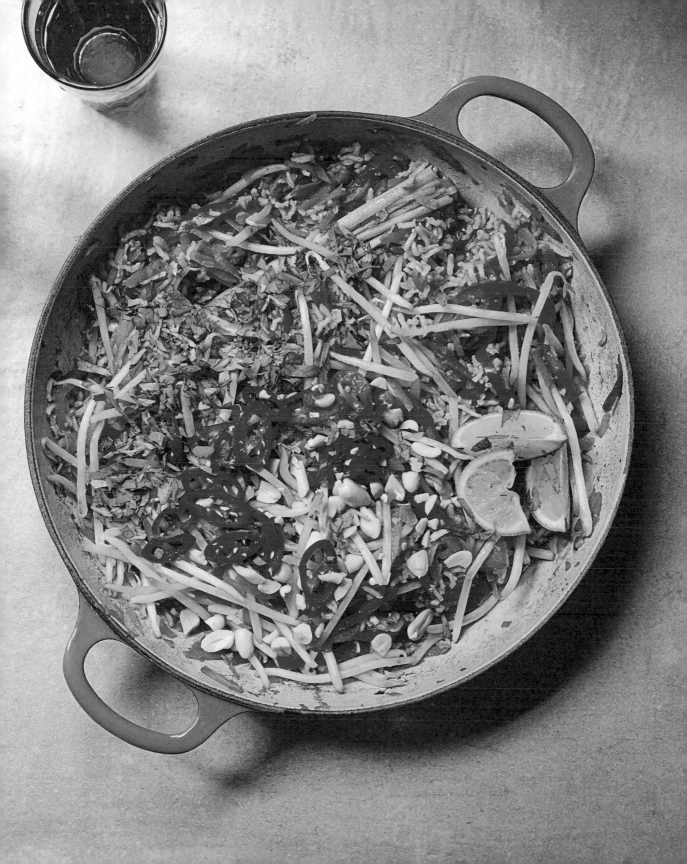

This is a take on *baghali polo*, a luxurious buttery Persian rice dish with dill and saffron. The delicious flavours sing through the wonderful wholegrains and peas and the saffron butter is a nod to the inspiration behind this recipe.

Broad Bean, Pea and Dill Rice

1 Put the oil, rice, beans and peas into a lidded casserole dish or sauté pan over a medium heat. Crumble in the stock cube. Pour over the boiling water, season with salt and pepper and stir.

2 Cover and simmer for 30 minutes, until the rice is almost tender and the water has almost all been absorbed.

3 Stir in the dill, parsley and ripe tomatoes, re-cover and cook for a further 5 minutes.

4 Mix the saffron and butter together in a small bowl.

5 Remove the pan from the heat, dot the rice all over with the saffron butter, re-cover and leave to stand for 5 minutes to allow the saffron butter to melt. Serve straight away with extra chopped dill.

PREP 5 MINUTES/COOK 40 MINUTES

1 tbsp extra-virgin olive oil
100g brown rice, rinsed
160g broad beans (fresh or frozen)
160g peas (fresh or frozen)
1 vegetable stock cube
300ml boiling water
20g fresh dill, chopped, plus extra to serve
20g fresh flat-leaf parsley, chopped
160g ripe tomatoes, diced
pinch of saffron strands
20g unsalted butter, softened
sea salt and freshly ground black pepper

Cook's tip

You can use extra olive oil to serve, instead of the saffron butter, if you prefer it to be fully plant-based.

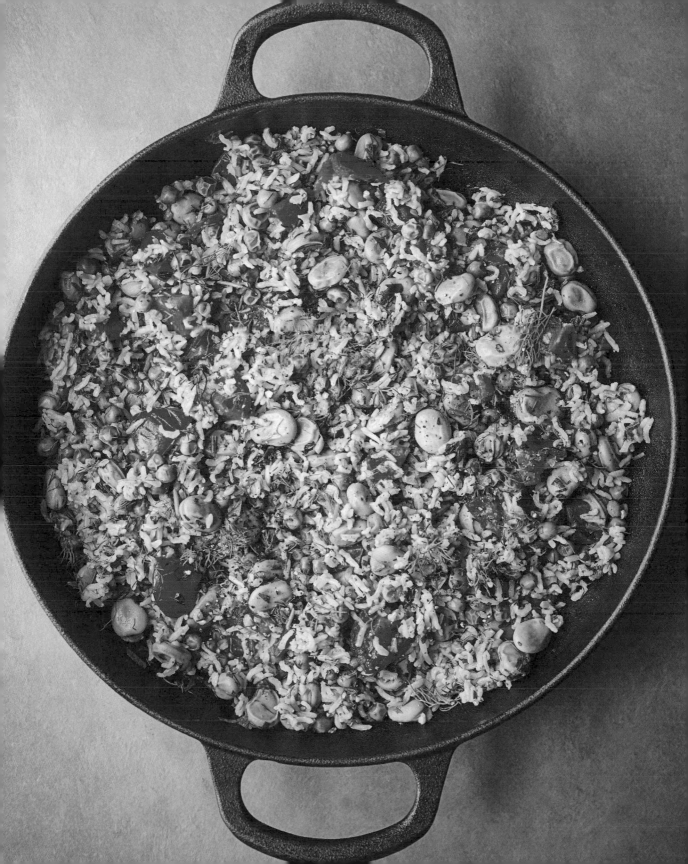

The classic Jamaican flavours of ginger, allspice and cinnamon, with the punchy heat of Scotch bonnet, are a firm favourite and this easy rice and pea dish delivers those beautiful combinations.

Jamaican-style Rice and Peas

1 Heat the coconut oil in a small casserole dish over a medium heat. Stir in the rice and coat with the oil. Add the garlic, ginger, spring onions and pepper and fry for 2–3 minutes.

2 Add the black-eyed peas, bay leaf and spices and crumble in the stock cube. Season and pour over the boiling water. Cover and simmer gently for 30–35 minutes until the rice is tender.

3 Meanwhile, toss all the slaw ingredients together in a bowl, season to taste and set aside to infuse.

4 Remove the Scotch bonnet from the rice and serve the rice with the slaw.

Cook's tip

You can omit the Scotch bonnet or use a milder spice if you prefer less heat.

Variation

Try using kidney beans, and adding sliced chicken to the rice while it cooks.

PREP 10 MINUTES / COOK 35 MINUTES

2 tbsp coconut oil

100g brown rice, rinsed

2 garlic cloves, grated

15g piece of root ginger (about 1.5cm), grated

60g spring onions (about 4), sliced

160g deseeded green pepper (about 1 large), diced

400g tin black-eyed peas, drained and rinsed

1 bay leaf

1 cinnamon stick

1 Scotch bonnet chilli, halved

1 tsp fennel seeds

½ tsp ground allspice

1 vegetable stock cube

300ml boiling water

sea salt and freshly ground black pepper

FOR THE SLAW

20g fresh coriander, leaves and stalks finely chopped

160g red cabbage (about ¼), finely shredded

100g peeled and grated carrot (about 1)

60g finely diced, peeled apple

finely grated zest and juice of 1 lime

2 tbsp extra-virgin olive oil

I tend to make this dish when I have a little more time on my hands, because I find the gentle and rhythmic action of pouring in stock, while watching and listening to the risotto cook, quite therapeutic.

Spinach and Watercress Risotto

1 Heat the oil in a sauté pan over a low heat, add the celery, parsley stalks and leeks and fry gently for 5 minutes until softened.

2 Add the rice and stir it in the hot oil for a minute to toast the grains, then add the wine and stir until the wine is absorbed (about 2 minutes).

3 Mix the stock cube and boiling water in a heatproof jug. Add the stock to the rice a little at a time, stirring constantly, allowing each addition to absorb before adding more.

4 After 16–18 minutes, once almost all the stock has been added, stir in the watercress, spinach and parsley leaves and allow to wilt. Season well.

5 Add the last bit of stock and the cheese, stir and remove from the heat. Leave to stand for 3–4 minutes, then serve.

PREP 10 MINUTES/COOK 30 MINUTES

2 tbsp extra-virgin olive oil
100g celery (1–2 stalks), finely diced
15g fresh flat-leaf parsley, leaves and stalks finely chopped
160g leeks (1 large or 2 small), finely diced
120g carnaroli or arborio risotto rice
150ml dry white wine
1 vegetable stock cube
700ml boiling water
160g watercress, roughly chopped
160g spinach, roughly torn
60g finely grated Parmesan or pecorino cheese
sea salt and freshly ground black pepper

Variation

Try adding asparagus, broad beans or even peas as an alternative to the watercress.

Whole Grains

I love a classic risotto but this twist, made with pearl barley instead of risotto rice, is just as satisfying and makes for a wonderfully balanced springtime dish.

Pearl Barley, Mint and Asparagus Risotto

1 Heat the oil in a lidded sauté pan over a low to medium heat and add the onion, celery and fennel, frying gently for 5 minutes until softened.

2 Add the pearl barley and toast in the pan for a minute, then add the stock and lemon zest.

3 Season well, cover and simmer for 40 minutes until the grains are nearly tender. The mixture should be a little soupy, just like a risotto made with rice.

4 Add the asparagus and mint and cook for a further 2 minutes until the asparagus is tender. Remove from the heat, add the Parmesan and a good squeeze of lemon juice and serve.

PREP 10 MINUTES / COOK 50 MINUTES

2 tbsp extra-virgin olive oil
100g onion (about 1 small), finely chopped
160g celery (3–4 stalks), finely chopped
160g fennel (about 1 small bulb), finely chopped
120g pearl barley
1 vegetable stock cube dissolved in 500ml boiling water
finely grated zest and juice of 1 lemon
160g asparagus spears, sliced into 2cm pieces
1 tbsp finely chopped fresh mint
3 tbsp finely grated Parmesan cheese
sea salt and freshly ground black pepper

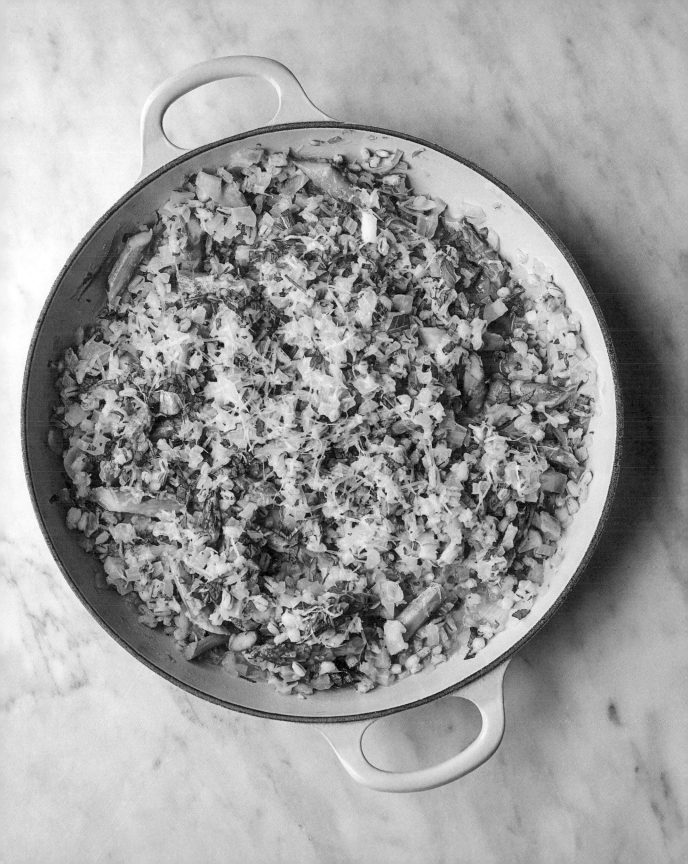

This rich tomato and rice dish, with gorgeous cardamom, cloves, cinnamon and bay, is exactly how a pilau should be. It's a joy to eat and share.

Ginger and Tomato Pilau

1 Heat the oil in a lidded casserole dish or sauté pan over a medium heat, add the ginger, garlic and curry leaves and fry for a minute or two until fragrant.

2 Add the rice and spices and allow to coat in the oil for a minute.

3 Add the tomatoes, stock, season with salt and pepper, cover and simmer for 30 minutes.

4 Add the carrot and spring greens. Re-cover and cook for a further 3–4 minutes until the greens are tender and juicy.

5 Remove from the heat and stand, covered, for 5 minutes, then serve scattered with the coriander and cashews.

Cook's tip

Don't worry if you can't find curry leaves; the rest of the spices carry a lot of flavour regardless. To make it quicker, you can even simply use 2 teaspoons garam masala.

PREP 15 MINUTES/COOK 40 MINUTES

2 tbsp extra-virgin olive oil

15g piece of root ginger (about 1.5cm), peeled and grated

3 garlic cloves, grated

15 fresh curry leaves

100g brown basmati rice, rinsed

1 cinnamon stick

2 cloves

2 cardamom pods, bashed

1 bay leaf

1 green chilli, sliced in half

400g tin chopped tomatoes

½ vegetable stock cube dissolved in 300ml boiling water

160g carrots (1 large or 2 small), grated

160g spring greens, shredded

sea salt and freshly ground black pepper

TO SERVE

15g fresh coriander, leaves and stalks finely chopped

20g cashews, chopped

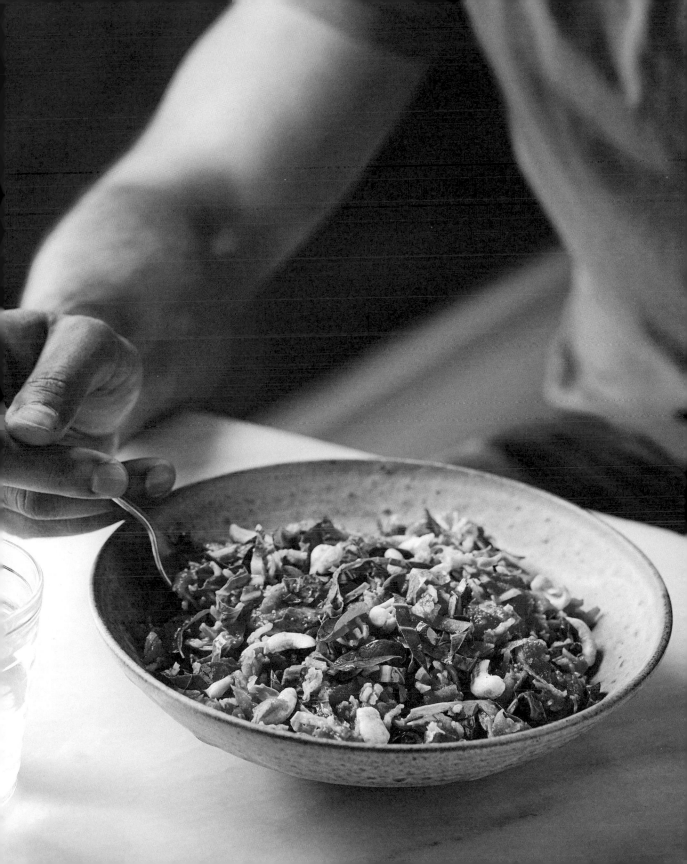

This simple paella dish is a delight to eat and cook. The addition of leek and artichokes brings a wonderful sweetness and they merge with the smoky paprika really well.

Leek, Artichoke and Prawn Paella

1 Heat the oil in a sauté pan or shallow casserole dish over a medium heat, add the leeks and courgettes and fry for 5 minutes until softened and lightly golden.

2 Add the paprika and bay leaf, then stir in the rice and toast for a minute.

3 Add the tomatoes, saffron and stock, season well and cook for 15 minutes, until the rice is tender and the stock is almost all absorbed (no need to stir).

4 Stir in the artichokes and prawns and cover. Cook for 4–5 minutes until the prawns are pink all over.

5 Uncover and cook for another minute, then remove from the heat and serve scattered with parsley and lemon wedges to squeeze over.

PREP 15 MINUTES/COOK 25 MINUTES

2 tbsp extra-virgin olive oil
160g leeks (1 large or 2 small), chopped
160g courgettes (1–2), sliced into 5cm-long batons
2 tsp smoked paprika
1 bay leaf
100g paella rice
about 100g ripe tomatoes, finely chopped
good pinch of saffron strands
1 vegetable stock cube dissolved in 500ml boiling water
160g roast artichoke hearts (from a jar), drained, and sliced if large
6–8 raw, shell-on king prawns
sea salt and freshly ground black pepper

TO SERVE

15g fresh flat-leaf parsley, leaves and stalks finely chopped
1 lemon, cut into wedges

Variation

This works well without the prawns if you want to make it vegetarian. You could also use any chunks of white fish, such as bream or bass.

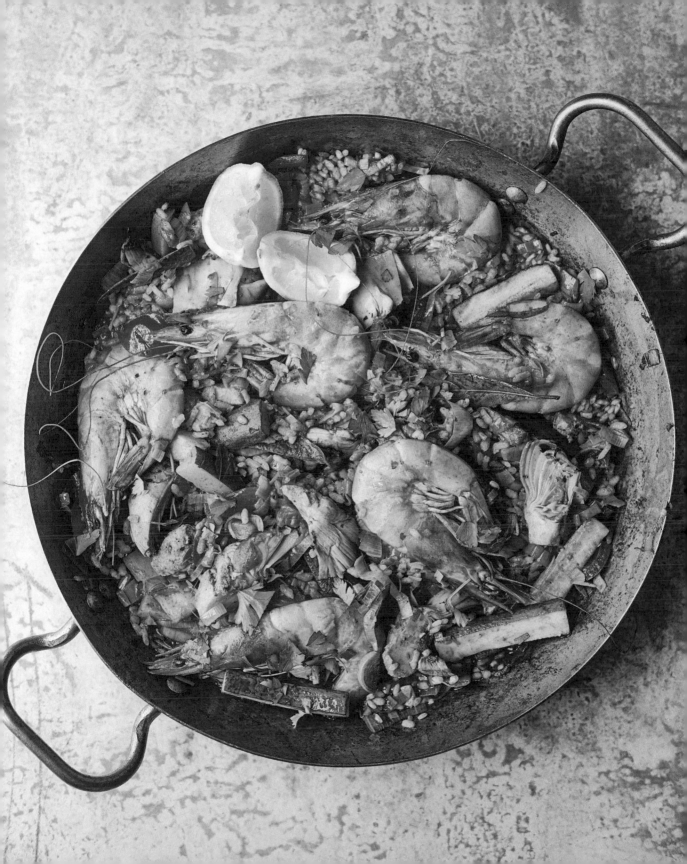

Tray
Bakes

When I've got a cauliflower and I'm lost for inspiration, I turn to this simple recipe that uses up every part of it. It's delicious, filling and super easy.

Massaman Cauliflower

1 Preheat the oven to 200°C/180°C fan/gas 6.

2 Remove the base of the cauliflower. Roughly chop the leaves and put in a roasting tray with the tomatoes, chilli, garlic and lime zest.

3 Cut the cauliflower into 4 wedges, smear with the massaman paste and snuggle them into the greens and tomatoes in the pan. Season with salt and pepper, squeeze over the lime juice and drizzle with the soy sauce.

4 Roast in the oven for 15 minutes then remove, baste the cauliflower with the cooking juices, add the lentils, stir and roast for a further 15 minutes until the cauliflower is roasted, golden and tender.

5 Remove from the oven and serve scattered with the coriander leaves, and lime wedges for squeezing.

PREP 10 MINUTES / COOK 30 MINUTES

750g cauliflower (about 1 cauliflower), with leaves
200g cherry tomatoes, halved
1 red chilli, finely chopped
2 garlic cloves, grated
grated zest and juice of 1 lime, plus extra wedges to serve
4 tsp massaman paste (from a jar)
2 tbsp soy sauce
400g tin green lentils, drained and rinsed
sea salt and freshly ground black pepper
25g fresh coriander leaves, to serve

Variation

Try this with tinned chickpeas for a twist, and it also works well with harissa paste.

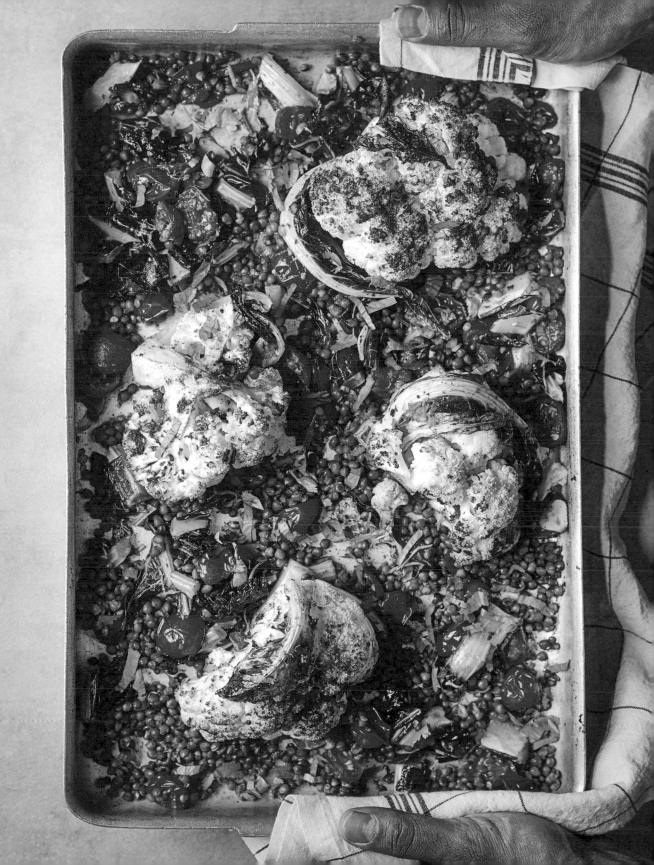

Trust me with the pineapple in this one – the sweet and spicy flavours are well matched and it's a great way of experimenting with new ingredients.

Smoky Glazed Pepper and Prawn Tacos with Caramelised Pineapple

1 Preheat the grill to high. Put the prawns, pepper and pineapple in a baking tray and smother in the oil, spices, soy sauce and maple syrup.

2 Grill for 4–5 minutes until the prawn tails catch and the flesh is cooked.

3 Remove the tray, pick out the prawns and set aside. Cook the vegetables under the grill for 5 minutes more until caramelised.

4 Remove the tray, return the prawns, scatter with the coriander and garnish with the lime zest and juice. Season with salt and pepper.

5 Serve on corn tacos with the avocado, more lime juice and the rest of the coriander.

Variation

Try making this with edamame beans instead of prawns for a plant-based meal.

PREP 10 MINUTES/COOK 10 MINUTES

200g raw shelled tiger or king prawns, deveined, tails on

160g deseeded red pepper (1 large), thinly sliced

160g skinned, cored pineapple, cut into 2cm chunks

2 tbsp extra-virgin olive oil

1 tsp smoked paprika

½ tsp ground cumin

1 tbsp soy sauce

1 tbsp maple syrup

20g fresh coriander, leaves torn

grated zest and juice of 1 lime

160g peeled and stoned avocado (1 large or 2 small), diced

sea salt and freshly ground black pepper

4–6 soft corn tacos, to serve

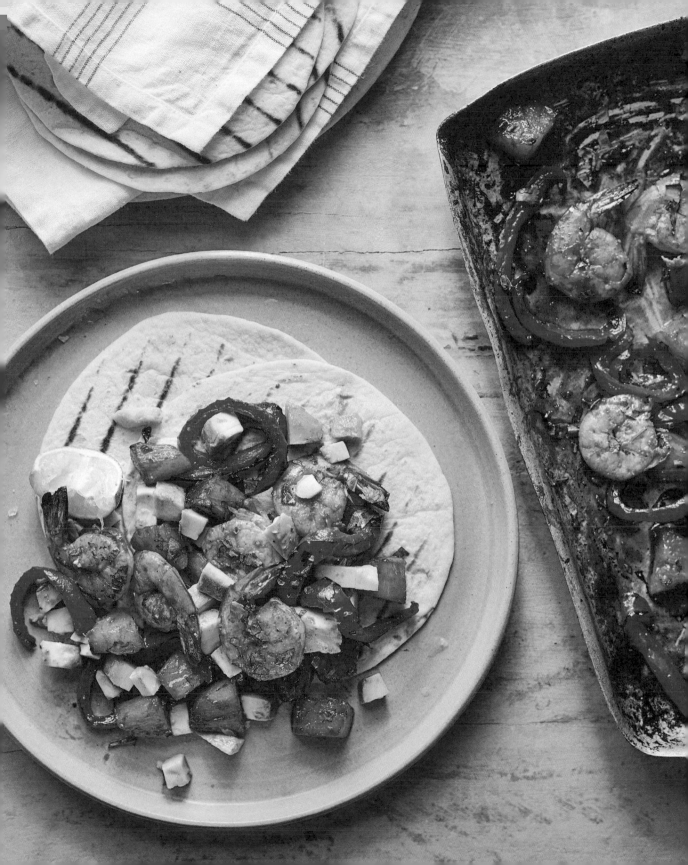

The beautiful intensity of mushrooms in this delicious one-tray dish is brought out by baking them and using soy sauce.

Spicy Garlic Mushrooms with Pomegranate

1 Preheat the oven to 220°C/200°C fan/gas 7.

2 Put the mushrooms in a roasting tray with the onions and garlic. Add the spices, soy sauce and olive oil, toss together and season with salt and pepper.

3 Roast in the oven for about 20–25 minutes, tossing once or twice, until the mushrooms and onions are tender and golden.

4 Remove from the oven, toss with the watercress and serve with a scattering of pomegranate seeds and a drizzle more oil.

PREP 10 MINUTES/COOK 25 MINUTES

200g mixed mushrooms (such as shiitake, oyster, portobello), roughly ripped up

160g red onion (about 1 medium), sliced into thin wedges

2 garlic cloves, thinly sliced

1 tsp cumin seeds or ground cumin

1 tsp smoked sweet paprika

good pinch of dried chilli flakes

1 tbsp soy sauce

2 tbsp extra-virgin olive oil, plus extra for drizzling

160g watercress, roughly torn

sea salt and freshly ground black pepper

50g pomegranate seeds, to serve

Variation

Try adding 2 thinly sliced chicken thighs or cooked black lentils to the tray if you want a more filling meal.

The addition of pomegranate molasses to the harissa balances the heat of the fiery paste and helps makes a gorgeous, easy dish look as spectacular as it tastes.

Harissa Fennel, Aubergine and Chickpeas

1 Preheat the oven to 200°C/180°C fan/gas 6.

2 Mix the harissa and sun-dried tomato paste with the oil and pomegranate molasses. Smother the aubergine, fennel and chickpeas with the mixture in a roasting tray and season with salt and pepper.

3 Roast in the oven for 30 minutes, turning the vegetables and chickpeas once or twice, until the aubergine is really tender. Add the pine nuts for the last 10 minutes of cooking to toast them.

4 Remove from the oven, spoon onto a platter, scatter with the preserved lemon and dill or fennel fronds to serve.

PREP 10–15 MINUTES/COOK 30 MINUTES

1 tbsp harissa paste

1 tbsp sun-dried tomato paste

3 tbsp extra-virgin olive oil

1 tbsp pomegranate molasses

200g aubergine (about 1 large), cut into chunky 2cm batons

160g fennel (about 1 small bulb), cut into thin wedges

400g tin chickpeas, drained and rinsed

20g pine nuts

sea salt and freshly ground black pepper

TO SERVE

1 preserved lemon, rind thinly sliced (flesh discarded)

10g picked fresh dill or fennel fronds

Cook's tip

You can just use a squeeze of lemon juice instead of the preserved lemon, if you prefer.

Tray Bakes

Many of us can't quite picture how to use celeriac in a dish. This method of roasting it with punchy spices brings out its incredible flavour and the addition of citrus balances the meal.

Baked, Spiced Celeriac with Hummus and Pomelo

1 Preheat the oven to 200°C/180°C fan/gas 6.

2 Toss the celeriac and chickpeas in a roasting tray with the spices, oregano and oil and season well.

3 Roast in the oven for 30 minutes, stirring once, until the celeriac is tender. Discard the cinnamon stick and tip the celeriac and chickpeas into a bowl.

4 Segment the pomelo, toss these, along with the rocket, through the baked celeriac and chickpeas with another drizzle of olive oil.

5 Mix the hummus with the harissa or paprika and dollop onto two plates. Top with the baked celeriac mix.

Variation

If you can't get hold of a pomelo, this dish would be just as delicious using ruby grapefruit or orange segments instead.

PREP 10 MINUTES/COOK 30 MINUTES

200g peeled celeriac, cut into 1.5cm cubes
400g tin chickpeas, drained and rinsed
3 cardamom pods, cracked
1 cinnamon stick
¼ tsp ground allspice
6 black peppercorns, roughly crushed
1 tsp cumin seeds
1 tsp dried chilli flakes
2 tsp dried oregano
2 tbsp extra-virgin olive oil, plus extra for drizzling
250g pomelo
50g wild rocket leaves
200g hummus
2 tsp rose harissa paste or 1 tsp hot smoked paprika
sea salt and freshly ground black pepper

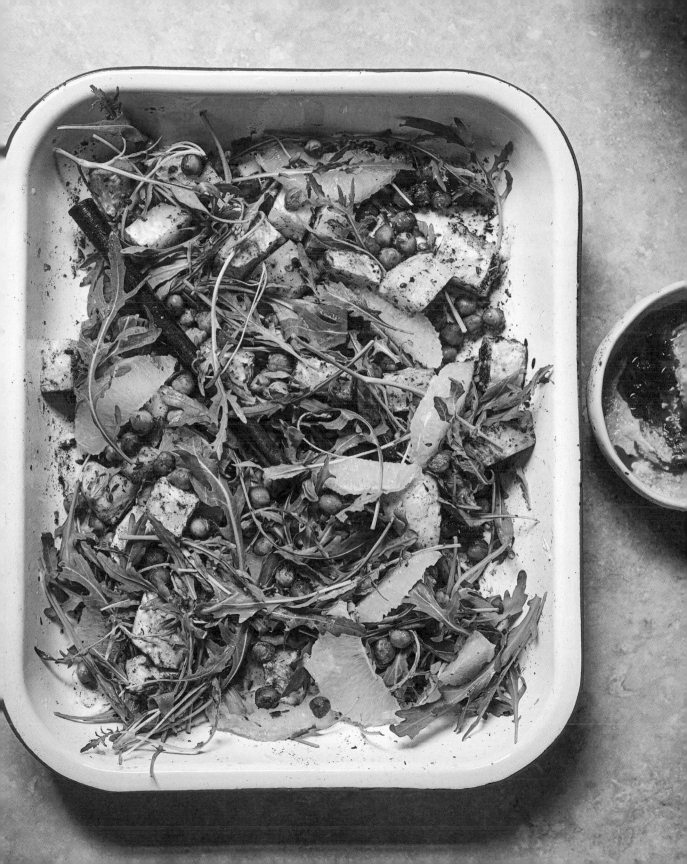

An exotic mix of flavours inspired by Sri Lankan cuisine. I love serving this with simple fragrant rice, but the chickpeas bulk it up into a satiating meal on its own.

Roasted Masala Chickpeas with Green Bean Sambol

1 Preheat the oven to 200°C/180°C fan/gas 6.

2 Toss the chickpeas, cashews, parsley stalks and green beans in the coconut oil and spices in a roasting tray. Season well with salt and pepper.

3 Roast in the oven for 10–15 minutes, until the beans are tender and the chickpeas are golden.

4 Remove from the oven and toss with the parsley, tomatoes, coconut, lime zest and juice and shallot. Season again and serve.

Variation

You can also use freshly podded peas or mangetout instead of green beans.

PREP 5 MINUTES/COOK 15 MINUTES

400g tin chickpeas, drained and rinsed
30g cashews, chopped
60g fresh flat-leaf parsley, finely chopped, and stalks
160g green beans
1 tbsp coconut oil
2 tsp Sri Lankan curry powder or garam masala
½ tsp ground cinnamon
pinch of dried chilli flakes
200g cherry tomatoes, chopped
60g freshly grated coconut (or dry desiccated coconut)
finely grated zest and juice of 1 lime
90g banana shallot (about 1), thinly sliced
sea salt and freshly ground black pepper

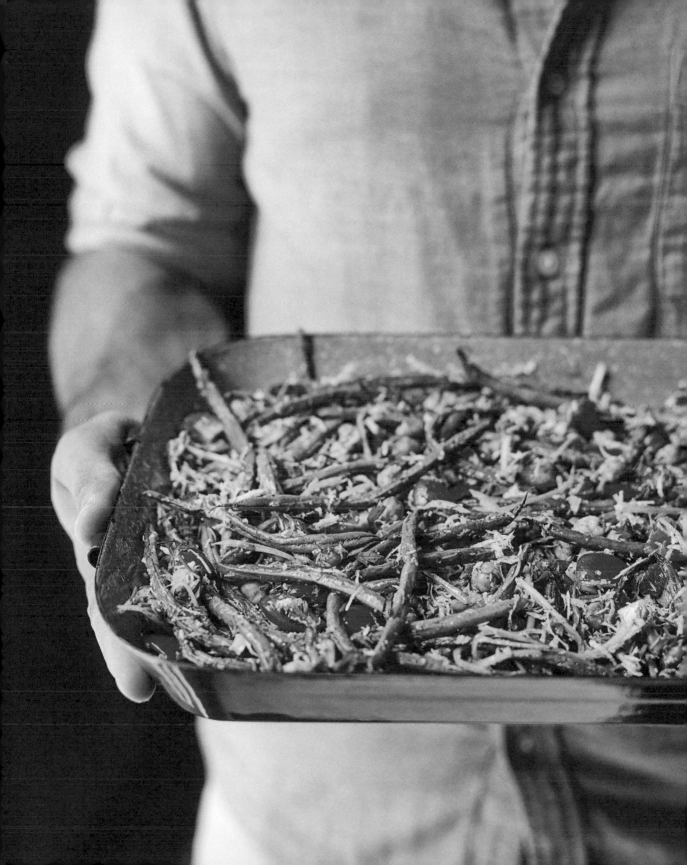

The simplicity of the herbs, matched with the crunch of roasted breadcrumbs and the vibrant broccoli makes this a spectacular dish.

Herb-baked Aubergine with Tenderstem Broccoli

1 Preheat the oven to 200°C/180°C fan/gas 6.

2 Toss the aubergine with the oil, chilli, dried herbs and garlic in a roasting tray. Drizzle over the soy sauce and season with salt and pepper. Roast in the oven for 25 minutes.

3 Toss in the Tenderstem broccoli and beans, scatter with the breadcrumbs, drizzle with oil and roast for a further 10 minutes until the broccoli is just cooked.

4 Remove from the oven and toss with the parsley and a good squeeze of lemon juice. Add another drizzle of olive oil, check the seasoning and serve.

PREP 5 MINUTES/COOK 35 MINUTES

160g aubergine (about 1 large), cut into 2cm cubes

2 tbsp extra-virgin olive oil, plus extra for drizzling

½ tsp dried chilli flakes

2 tsp dried Herbes de Provence

4 garlic cloves, unpeeled

1 tbsp soy sauce

160g Tenderstem broccoli, roughly chopped

400g tin borlotti beans, drained and rinsed

2 tbsp white or brown fresh breadcrumbs

15g fresh flat-leaf parsley, chopped

½ lemon

sea salt and freshly ground black pepper

The combination of capers, pine nuts and balsamic vinegar is a sensational flavour enhancer for the tomatoes, and pairs beautifully with simple white fish.

Roast Sea Bass and Asparagus with Tomatoes and Capers

1 Preheat the oven to 200°C/180°C fan/gas 6.

2 Toss the asparagus with the tomatoes, capers, pine nuts and chilli flakes in a roasting tray. Drizzle with the vinegar and most of the oil and season well with salt and pepper. Roast in the oven for 15–20 minutes.

3 Add the spinach to the roasting tray, toss, and top with the fish fillets, skin side up. Season, drizzle with the rest of the oil and roast for a further 10–12 minutes until the fish is cooked.

4 Remove from the oven, scatter with the parsley and serve.

PREP 10 MINUTES/COOK 25–35 MINUTES

160g asparagus
200g ripe tomatoes, roughly chopped
2 tbsp capers, drained and rinsed
30g pine nuts
½ tsp dried chilli flakes
1 tbsp aged balsamic vinegar
2 tbsp extra-virgin olive oil
160g baby spinach, roughly chopped
2 x 175g sea bass fillets, skin scored
sea salt and freshly ground black pepper
20g fresh flat-leaf parsley, chopped, to serve

Variations

Try using a stronger green leaf such as kale or cavolo nero, and swap the bass for a different white fish, such as pollock or even hake.

The simplest yet most delicious tray bake, made with vibrant corn, smoky spices and sweet tarragon: a beautiful mix of flavours and super easy to achieve.

Black-eyed Peas with Sweetcorn, Tarragon and Paprika

1 Preheat the oven to 200°C/180°C fan/gas 6.

2 Toss the black-eyed peas with the sweetcorn and onions in a roasting tray. Drizzle all over with the oil, add the paprika, oregano and garlic and season with salt and pepper.

3 Roast in the oven for 20 minutes until the onions are golden and tender and the sweetcorn is just cooked through.

4 Remove from the oven and squeeze over the lemon juice.

5 Muddle the rocket and tarragon through the warm ingredients, toss to combine, drizzle over some more extra-virgin olive oil and serve.

PREP 5 MINUTES/COOK 20 MINUTES

400g tin black-eyed peas, drained and rinsed
160g fresh sweetcorn kernels (sliced off about 2 sweetcorn cobs)
160g red onion (about 1 medium), sliced into thin wedges
2 tbsp extra-virgin olive oil, plus extra to serve
1 tsp paprika
1 tsp dried oregano
4 garlic cloves, thinly sliced
juice of ½ lemon
100g wild rocket leaves
15g fresh tarragon leaves
sea salt and freshly ground black pepper

Variations

Try using basil leaves or sage if you can't find tarragon. And this dish works well with black beans or even beautiful beluga lentils in place of the black-eyed peas.

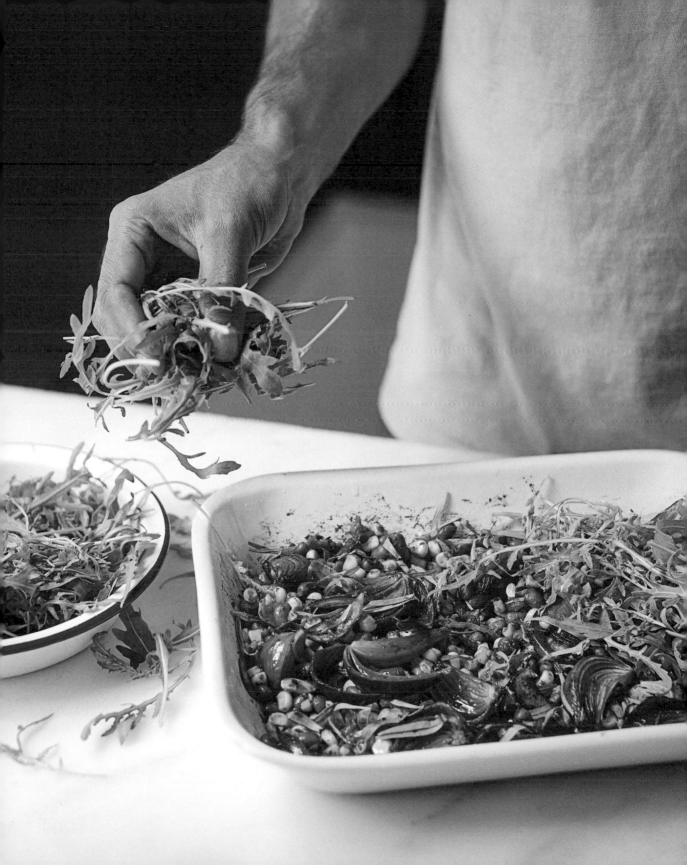

Tempeh is one of my favourite ingredients and I promise you that this dish will make you think differently about this wonderful ingredient if you're wary. The incredible sweet and rich spiciness of Korean gochujang paste, made with fermented soybeans, will also bring a new dimension to your home cooking.

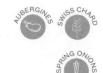

Gochujang Tempeh with Baby Aubergine and Sesame

1 Preheat the oven to 200°C/180°C fan/gas 6.

2 In a tray, mix the aubergine and tempeh with the gochujang paste, sesame oil, half the water and the pepper, then spread out. Bake in the oven for 20 minutes.

3 Turn the aubergine and tempeh and add the Swiss chard and spring onions. Toss with the sesame seeds and the rest of the water and roast for a further 10 minutes.

4 Remove from the oven and serve with a squeeze of lime juice.

PREP 10 MINUTES/COOK 30 MINUTES

200g baby aubergines (4–5), halved lengthways
200g tempeh, broken or cut into 2.5cm pieces
1 tbsp gochujang paste
2 tbsp sesame oil
4 tbsp boiling water
½ tsp freshly ground black pepper
160g Swiss chard, roughly chopped
160g spring onions (about 10–12), sliced
30g sesame seeds, plus extra to serve
juice of ½ lime

Cook's tips

If you can't get hold of baby aubergines, use large ones instead, cutting them into 1.5cm-wide batons. As an alternative to gochujang, use any chilli paste, with an added spoonful of miso paste or tomato purée for extra depth.

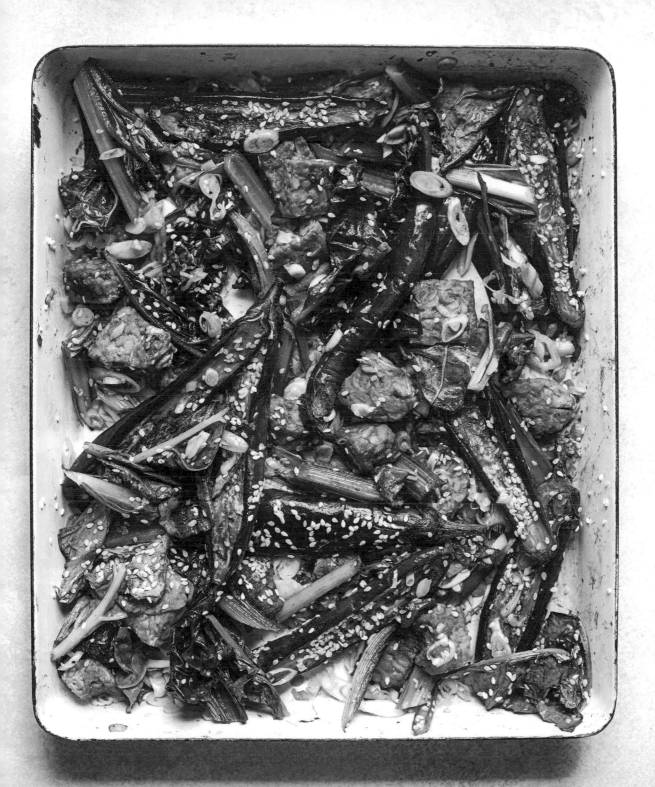

Roasting Brussels sprouts with a bit of soy sauce and sweetness is magical, but the dressing is what takes this dish to new levels.

Roasted Brassicas and Tofu with Chilli Miso Sauce

1 Preheat the oven to 200°C/180°C fan/gas 6.

2 Put the sprouts, broccoli, tofu, almonds and garlic in a roasting tray. Splash over the tamari or soy sauce and drizzle over the maple syrup and sesame oil. Scatter with the chilli flakes, season with black pepper and toss to coat.

3 Roast in the oven for 30 minutes, turning halfway through cooking, until golden and lightly charred.

4 Whisk all the ingredients for the dressing together in a bowl and set aside.

5 Remove the roasted brassicas and tofu from the oven and drizzle with the dressing to serve.

PREP 20 MINUTES/COOK 30 MINUTES

160g Brussels sprouts, quartered
160g purple-sprouting broccoli
200g firm tofu, cut into 2cm chunks
60g almonds, roughly chopped
3 garlic cloves, thinly sliced
1 tbsp tamari or soy sauce
1 tbsp maple syrup
1 tbsp sesame oil
pinch of dried chilli flakes
freshly ground black pepper

FOR THE DRESSING
2 tsp white miso paste
juice of 1 lemon
2 tbsp tahini
1 tsp dried chilli flakes
½ tsp freshly ground black pepper
60ml boiling water

Variation
Use edamame beans if you're not a fan of tofu.

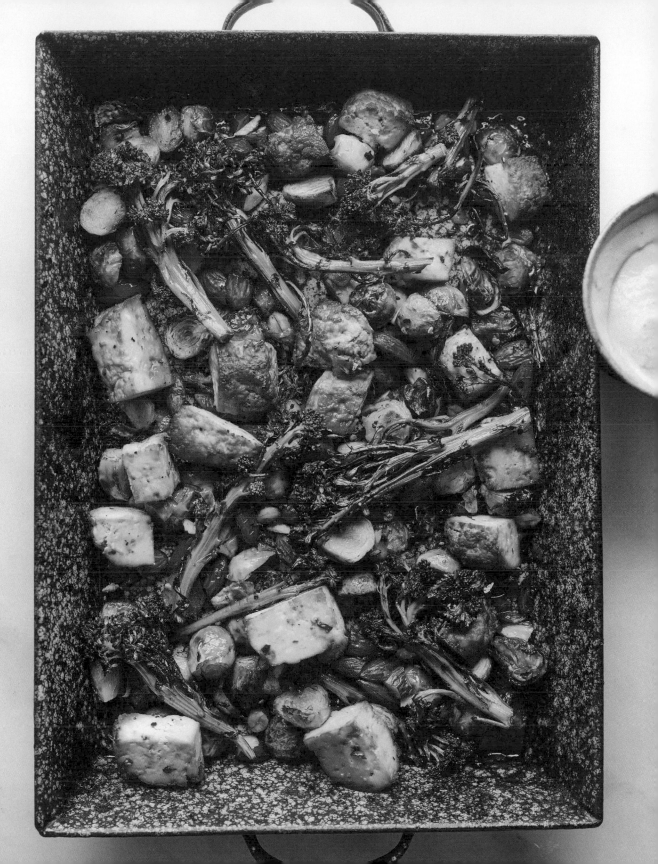

The combination of fennel, oregano and the clean taste of fresh sea bass is divine. This simple midweek meal is my go-to option when I fancy something a bit more luxurious but lack the time to create a decadent meal.

Baked Sea Bass Fillets with Fennel, Oregano and Lentils

1 Preheat the oven to 190°C/170°C fan/gas 5.

2 Put the broccoli, leeks and lemon slices in a roasting tray, add the oregano and spices, drizzle over half the oil and toss. Season and roast in the oven for 15 minutes.

3 Add the lentils to the roasting tray, stir, increase the oven temperature to 220°C/200°C fan/gas 7 and place the sea bass fillets on top, skin side up. Season the fish and drizzle with a little more of the oil.

4 Roast in the oven for 10–12 minutes more, until the fish is just cooked.

5 Remove from the oven and serve with a squeeze of lemon juice and the basil leaves scattered over.

PREP 10 MINUTES/COOK 25–30 MINUTES

160g purple-sprouting broccoli
160g baby leeks, halved lengthways
1 lemon, half sliced and half juiced
1 tsp dried oregano
1 tsp fennel seeds
1 tsp dried chilli flakes
2 tbsp extra-virgin olive oil
200g cooked puy lentils (from a tin or packet)
2 x 150g sea bass fillets, skin scored
sea salt and freshly ground black pepper
20g fresh basil leaves, torn, to serve

Variation

Use regular leeks if baby leeks are unavailable. The dish also works with Tenderstem broccoli or broccoli florets broken into 2cm pieces.

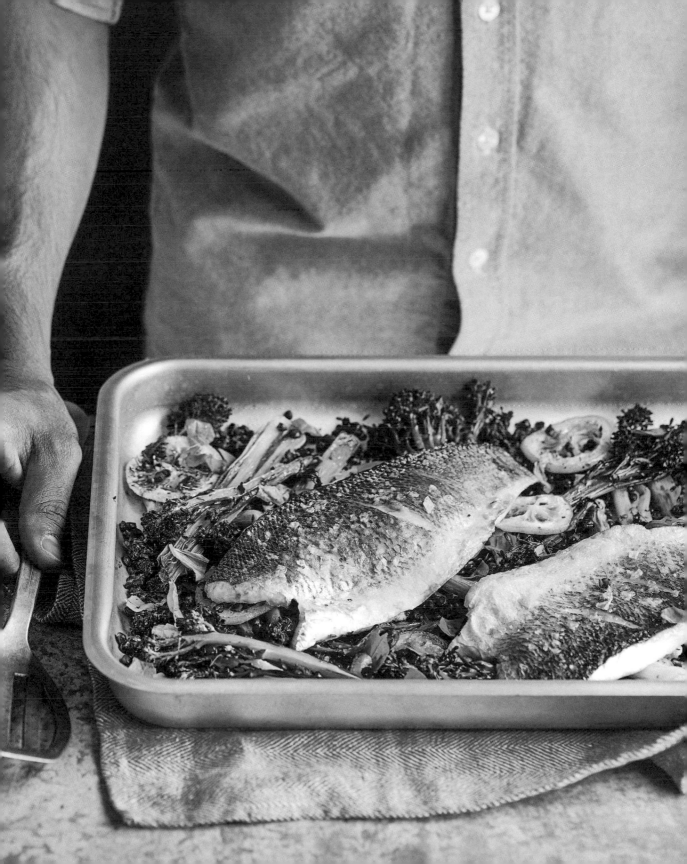

Cumin and cinnamon is such a powerful sweet and earthy spice combination: it transforms simple winter vegetables and this meal has a fantastic orchestra of flavours when cooked.

Cinnamon and Cumin Roasted Winter Vegetables with Baked Halloumi

1 Preheat the oven to 200°C/180°C fan/gas 6.

2 Tumble the onions, squash and sprouts into a roasting tray, smother with 1 tablespoon of the oil, plenty of salt and pepper and roast in the oven for 25 minutes.

3 Add the cumin, cinnamon, chilli flakes, sumac, pitta and halloumi to the vegetables in the tray, toss with the remaining tablespoon of oil and bake for a further 15 minutes until the pitta is crispy and golden and the halloumi is brown on the outside but soft and pillowy in the centre.

4 Remove from the oven and serve sprinkled with extra sumac, fresh mint and an extra drizzle of oil.

Variation

Omit the baked halloumi to make this completely plant-based if you wish.

PREP 10–15 MINUTES/COOK 40 MINUTES

160g red onion (about 1 medium), quartered

160g deseeded and skin-on butternut squash, sliced into 2cm-thick wedges

160g Brussels sprouts, halved

2 tbsp extra-virgin olive oil, plus extra for drizzling

2 tsp cumin seeds

½ tsp ground cinnamon

½ tsp dried chilli flakes

2 tsp sumac, plus extra to serve

2 wholemeal pittas, torn into chunks

200g halloumi, cut into 2cm-thick slices

sea salt and freshly ground black pepper

15g fresh mint leaves, chopped, to serve

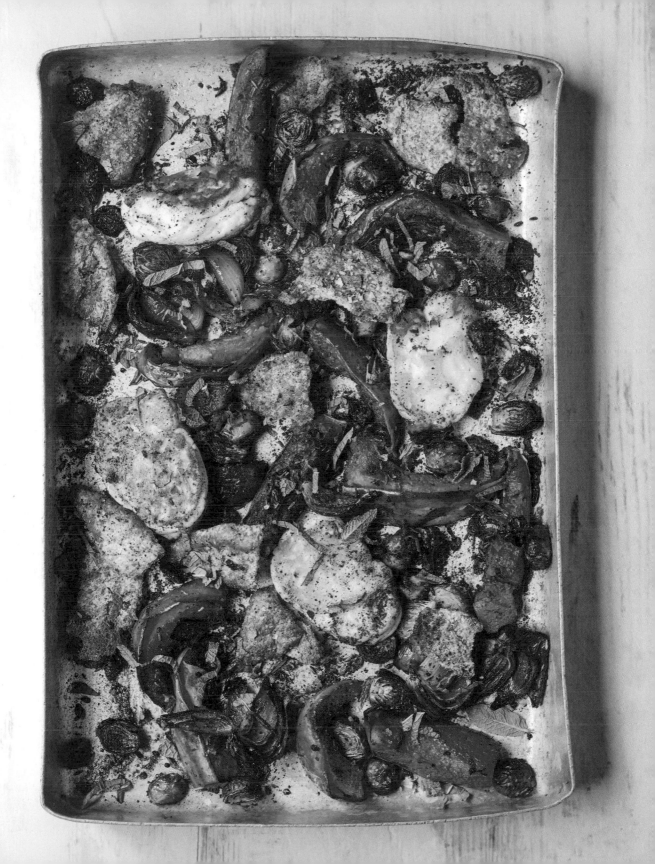

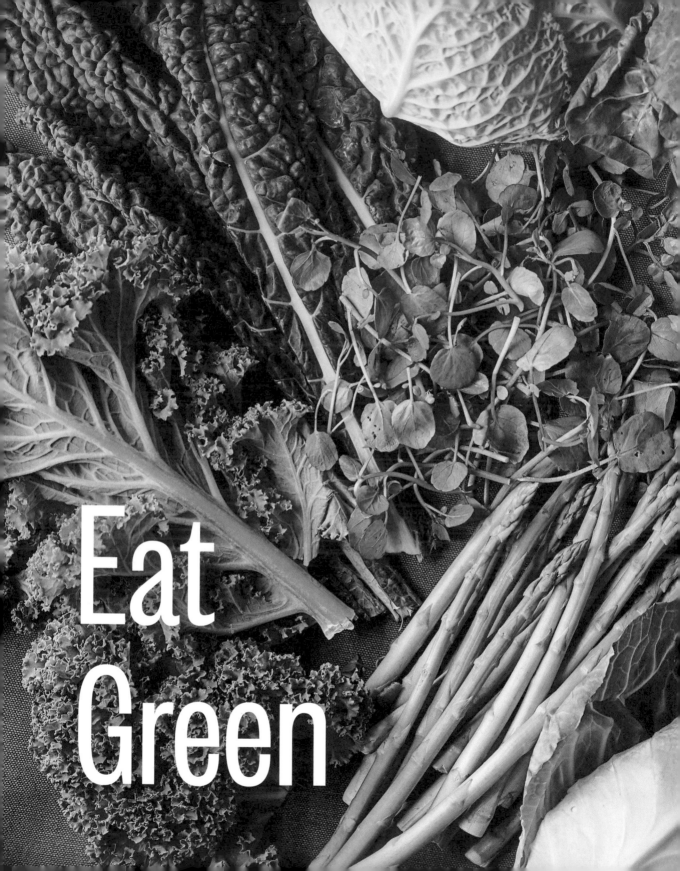

Eat
Green

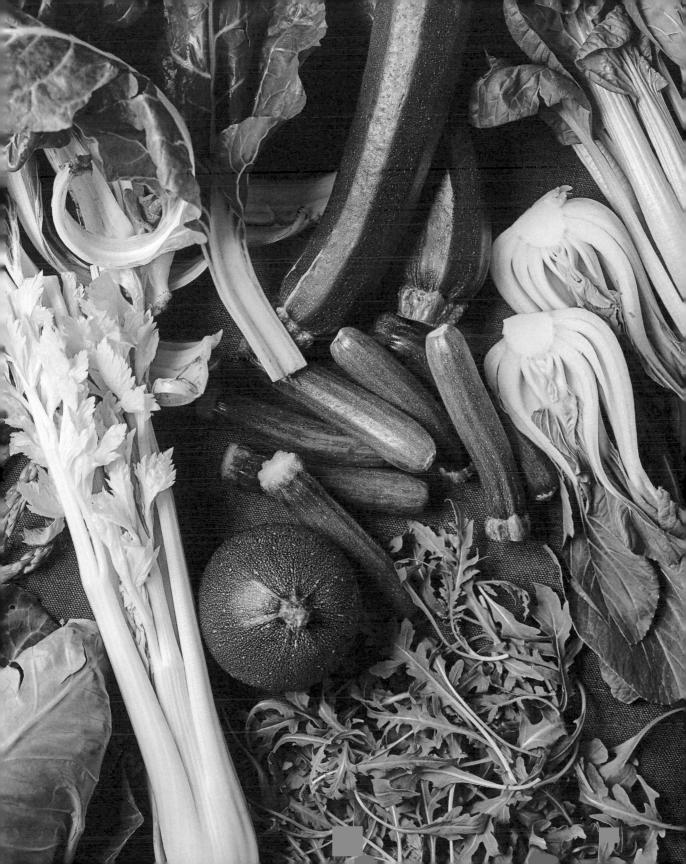

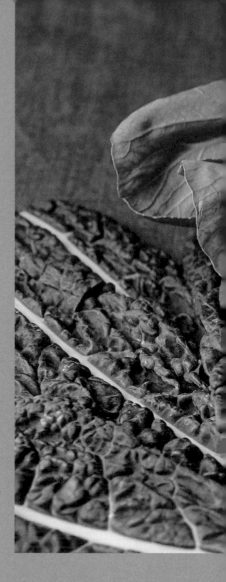

Greens such as spinach, Swiss chard and watercress can impact multiple systems in the body, including our brain function and heart health. Brassica vegetables, including broccoli, rocket, cabbage and Tuscan kale are particularly important to include in our diets. Also known as cruciferous vegetables, they release anti-cancer compounds, such as indoles and isothiocyanates, when chewed, bruised or chopped. As these compounds can be lost by overcooking, I tend to lightly cook or steam the ingredients to retain their health properties and have a portion most days. But, don't worry if some recipes call for greens to be cooked for a longer amount of time. You'll still receive a number of benefits from the fibre content of these vegetables that can benefit the microbiota, which has a direct role in modulating inflammation and improving your overall health.

Broccoli, collard greens and watercress in particular are some of those greens thought to be able to support detoxification by your organs as discussed on pages 34–6. Pak choi, watercress, Chinese cabbage and spinach are also high-nitrate vegetables that contribute to the production of vasoprotective nitric oxide, a chemical released in the blood vessel walls that relax the smooth muscle and lead to reduced blood pressure. This gives me yet another reason to prescribe daily greens, considering the global impact of raised blood pressure effecting 1 in every 6 people on the planet.

Some of the most exciting studies that I've come across relate to members of the cruciferous vegetable family (including broccoli, cabbage and cauliflower) and their impact on the expression of tumour suppressor genes that fight cancer cells. The nutrigenomic impact of green foods is

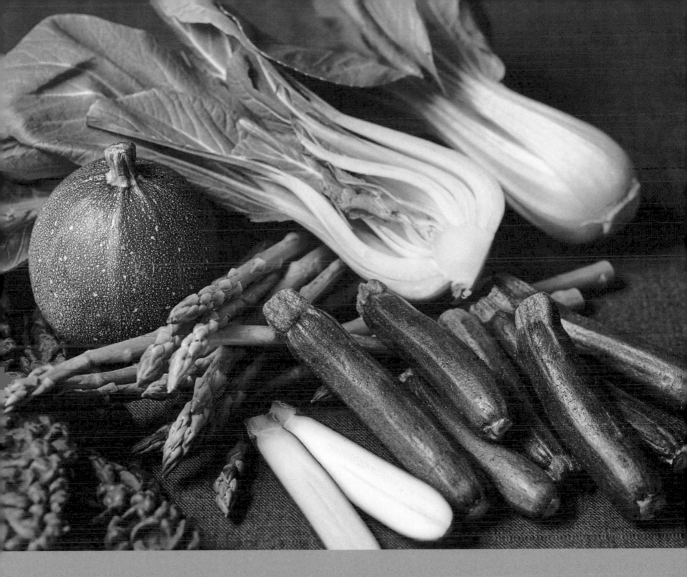

fascinating and may provide a plausible explanation as to why more greens in the diet are associated with lower rates of cancer overall. But more studies are needed to determine the definitive role of these foods. For now, I recommend their daily inclusion on your plates, as we already know enough about their role in health for me to suggest we should all be eating them regularly.

Across the wide spectrum of greens, they're also great sources of polyphenols, dietary antioxidants, and we recognise that consumption of fresh vegetables that are high in polyphenols is associated with a reduced risk of oxidative stress-induced disease including high blood pressure, diabetes and even mental health conditions.

Garam masala is a brilliant all-rounder spice blend and a couple of teaspoons transforms these simple vegetables in an instant.

Sweet Masala Charred Greens and Peanuts

1 Preheat the oven to 200°C/180°C fan/gas 6.

2 Toss the broccoli, spices, spring onions and peanuts in a roasting tray with the oil. Season well with salt and pepper and bake in the oven for 15 minutes.

3 Add the lentils and honey to the tray, toss and bake for a further 5 minutes.

4 Remove the tray from the oven, add the spinach and stir to wilt the leaves in the residual heat. Serve with the coriander and lemon juice.

Variation

Chickpeas would also work fantastically well with this dish instead of lentils.

PREP 10 MINUTES/COOK 20 MINUTES

160g Tenderstem broccoli, roughly chopped
2 tsp garam masala
½ tsp ground cinnamon
good pinch of red chilli powder
60g spring onions (about 4), chopped
60g unsalted peanuts, roughly chopped
2 tbsp extra-virgin olive oil, plus extra for drizzling
160g cooked black or brown lentils
1 tbsp honey
50g spinach, chopped
sea salt and freshly ground black pepper

TO SERVE
20g fresh coriander, torn
juice of ½ lemon

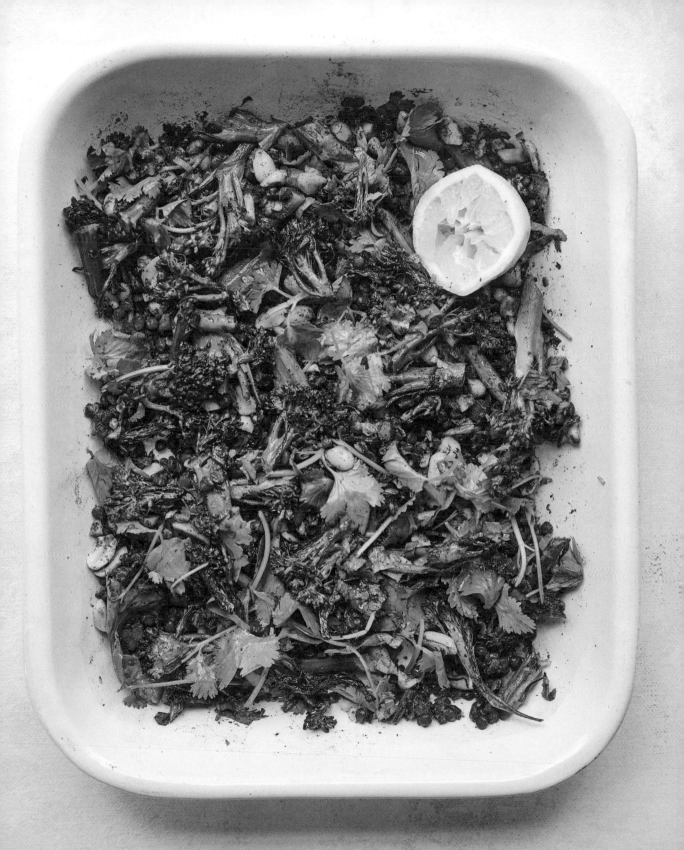

Sometimes, a store-bought jar of pesto or other paste adds all the flavour you need to make a beautifully balanced and speedy meal. I always have jarred flavour enhancers like this to hand.

Fennel, Leek and Beans with Basil Pesto

1 Preheat the oven to 190°C/170°C fan/gas 5.

2 Toss the fennel, beans and leeks in a roasting tray with the oil, pesto, lemon zest and juice and plenty of salt and pepper.

3 Roast in the oven for about 30–35 minutes.

4 Remove from the oven and serve the baked vegetables and beans scattered with chopped hazelnuts and basil leaves, with some warm crusty bread.

PREP 10 MINUTES/COOK 35 MINUTES

160g fennel (about 1 small bulb), sliced into thin wedges
400g tin flageolet beans, drained and rinsed
160g leeks (1 large or 2 small), sliced
2 tbsp extra-virgin olive oil
100g fresh basil pesto
finely grated zest and juice of 1 lemon
sea salt and freshly ground black pepper

TO SERVE
warm crusty bread
20g hazelnuts, chopped
10g fresh basil leaves

Variation

Try using a different pesto, such as red pepper pesto or even a homemade walnut version if you have time.

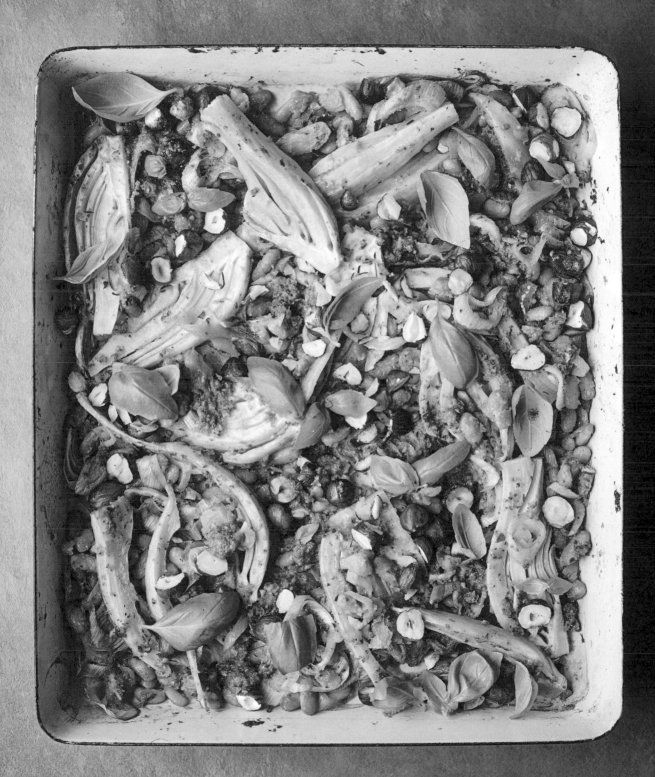

I'm taking liberties with the traditional use of a picada to add flavour to this simple meal. A picada is normally used to thicken Spanish stews and sauces, but it works fantastically here as a sort of salsa to dollop over your supper.

Spanish-style Beans with Marsala and an Almond Picada

1 Preheat the oven to 200°C/180°C fan/gas 6.

2 Toss the courgettes and tomatoes with the spices and bay leaf in a roasting tray. Drizzle with the oil, season well and roast in the oven for 20 minutes.

3 Add the marsala and beans to the roasting tray, toss and roast for 5–10 minutes, until the beans are warmed through and the vegetables are tender and roasted.

4 Meanwhile, pound the almonds, garlic and parsley in a large pestle and mortar. Add the bread and plenty of seasoning and pound to a paste, adding the oil a little at a time to a rough pesto-like mixture.

5 Remove the tray from the oven and serve the beans with dollops of picada.

PREP 20 MINUTES/COOK 25–30 MINUTES

160g baby courgettes, halved lengthways
200g ripe heritage tomatoes, halved or quartered
1 tsp sweet smoked paprika
1 tsp dried chilli flakes
1 bay leaf
2 tbsp extra-virgin olive oil
75ml marsala
400g tin cannellini beans, drained and rinsed
sea salt and freshly ground black pepper

FOR THE ALMOND PICADA
50g blanched almonds
1 garlic clove, peeled
25g fresh flat-leaf parsley
30g sourdough bread, torn into small pieces
5 tbsp extra-virgin olive oil

Cook's tip

Feel free to use a bullet blender to make the picada if you don't have a pestle and mortar. The marsala is really worth using in this dish but feel free to use a sweet wine or sherry instead if you prefer.

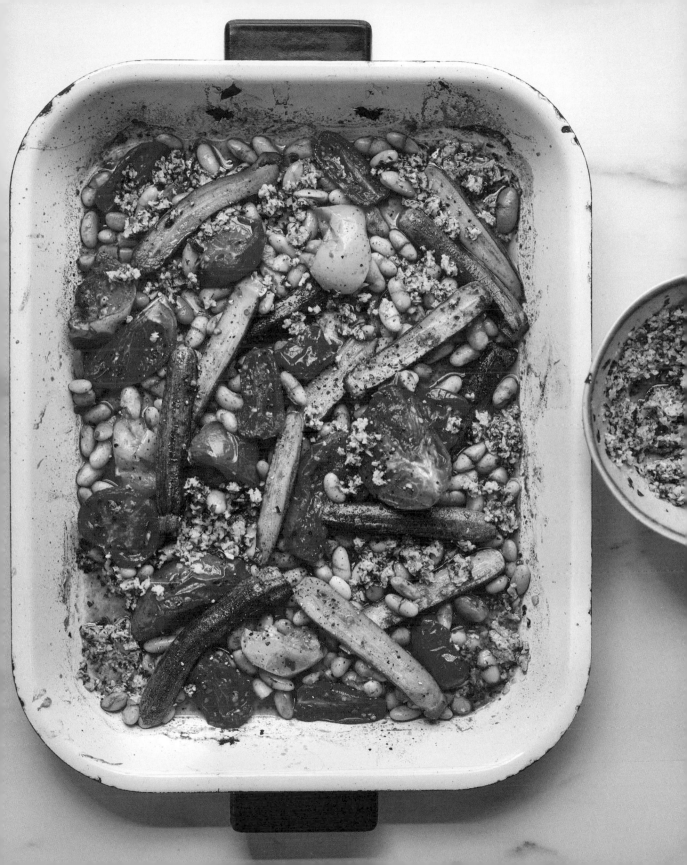

The fresh ginger and lemongrass really permeate through the delicious, fresh snapper. This is a midweek staple for me, and I always serve it with piles of greens.

Ginger and Lemongrass Snapper with Mangetout and Peas

1 Preheat the oven to 200°C/180°C fan/gas 6.

2 Whisk the ginger with the soy sauce, honey, fish sauce, sesame oil and the chilli in a small bowl.

3 Put the mangetout, peas and cabbage in a roasting tray, add the fish fillets skin side up and smother them with the ginger-soy mixture. Add the lemongrass and season the skin of the fish.

4 Cook for 8–10 minutes until the fish is cooked, the skin has crisped up and the vegetables are tender.

5 Garnish with pea shoots and spring onions and drizzle over the roasting pan juices to serve.

Variation

You could also use other firm fish such as bream or mackerel for this recipe.

PREP 15 MINUTES/COOK 10 MINUTES

50g piece of root ginger (about 5cm), grated
2 tbsp soy sauce
1 tbsp honey
2 tsp fish sauce
1 tbsp sesame oil
2 red chillies, thinly sliced
160g mangetout
160g fresh or frozen peas
160g Chinese cabbage or spring greens, thinly sliced
2 x 200g fillets of red snapper, skin scored
1 stick of lemongrass, bashed
sea salt and freshly ground black pepper

TO SERVE
50g pea shoots
45g spring onions (about 3), thinly sliced

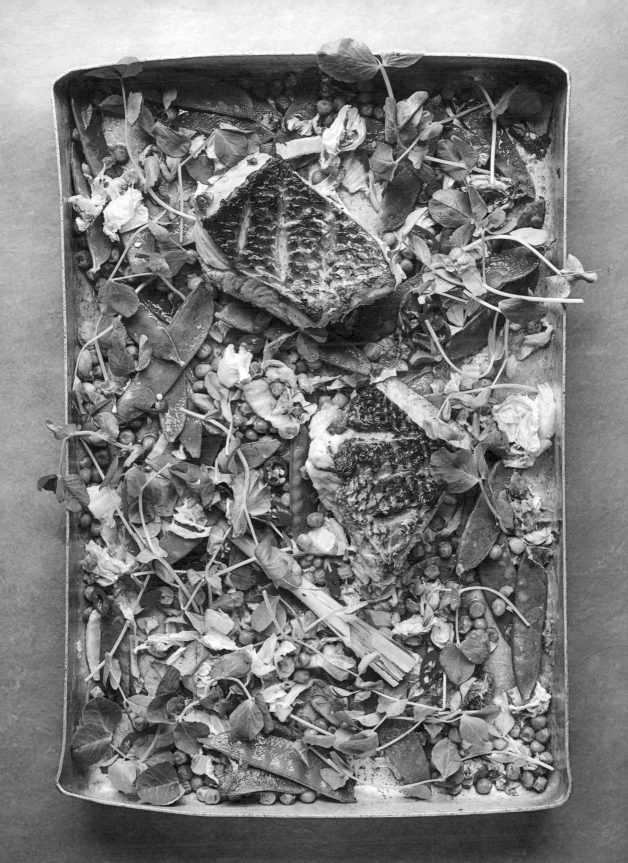

Curries

I had the privilege of visiting this beautiful country for a wedding and got the opportunity to stock up on authentic curry spice blends from the local markets. You can emulate the flavours using the list below – don't be put off by the amount of ingredients, it's well worth it for the experience!

Sri Lankan Polos Curry

1 Melt the coconut oil in a frying pan over a medium heat, add the red onion, ginger and garlic and fry gently for 5 minutes until softened.

2 Add all the spices and fry for a further minute. Add the cashews, tamarind and pandan (if using).

3 Stir in the jackfruit, coconut milk and tomatoes. Season with salt and pepper and simmer for 15 minutes until thickened and the jackfruit is collapsing slightly. Pull the jackfruit apart with two forks at the end of cooking, for better consistency.

4 Remove from the heat, stir in the desiccated coconut and scatter with the coriander leaves to serve.

Cook's tips

- Sri Lankan roast curry powder has a deep aromatic flavour, but if you can't get hold of it, use a medium curry powder.
- Pandan leaf grows in Southeast Asia and has an aromatic sweet flavour. It's available online but is not essential here.
- If you have time, dry-roast the desiccated coconut before cooking for more flavour.

PREP 10 MINUTES/COOK 25 MINUTES

1 tbsp coconut oil

100g red onion (about 1 small), thinly sliced

15g piece of root ginger (about 1.5cm), grated

4 garlic cloves, grated

1 tsp ground turmeric

1 tsp brown mustard seeds

4 cardamom pods, crushed

1 tsp cumin seeds

1 green chilli, finely chopped

1 cinnamon stick

2 tsp Sri Lankan curry powder (or mild curry powder)

60g cashews, roughly chopped

2 tsp tamarind paste

1 pandan leaf, cut into 3cm pieces (optional)

400g tin jackfruit, drained, rinsed and chopped

200ml coconut milk

400g tin chopped tomatoes

2 tbsp desiccated coconut

sea salt and freshly ground black pepper

15g fresh coriander leaves, chopped, to serve

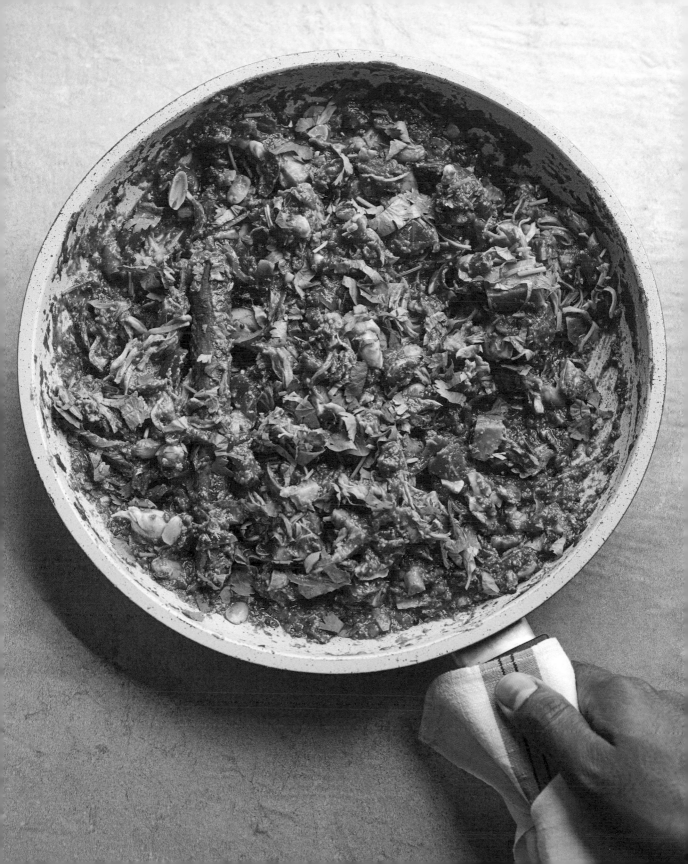

Once you've made this dish a couple of times, the prep will take you even less than 15 minutes. The spices work in effortless harmony to create a stunning and well-flavoured curry that is guaranteed to satisfy.

Butternut Korma

1 Heat the ghee or oil in a lidded sauté pan or casserole dish over a medium heat, add the onion and squash and fry for 5 minutes.

2 Add the garlic, ginger and the spices and cook for a further 5 minutes, then add the tomato purée and almonds.

3 Mix well, crumble in the stock cube, add the boiling water and season with salt and pepper. Cover and simmer for 10 minutes until the squash is tender.

4 Add the spinach and cook for a couple of minutes to wilt. Add the yoghurt and remove from the heat. Serve with the flaked almonds.

Cook's tips

To make this even quicker, try using 3 tablespoons of a simple curry paste in place of the ground spices if you're in a rush. Instead of ground almonds you could use the same amount of smooth almond nut butter.

PREP 15 MINUTES/COOK 25 MINUTES

3 tbsp ghee or coconut oil

200g onion (about 1 large), thinly sliced

350g deseeded butternut squash, skin on, cut into 3cm cubes

3 garlic cloves, grated

50g piece of root ginger (about 5cm), grated

2 tsp ground coriander

2 tsp ground cumin

¼ tsp ground turmeric

1 cinnamon stick

2 bay leaves

2 cloves

3 cardamom pods, cracked open

1 tbsp tomato purée

60g ground almonds

1 vegetable stock cube

500ml boiling water

160g spinach

150g unsweetened coconut yoghurt

sea salt and freshly ground black pepper

2 tbsp flaked almonds, to serve

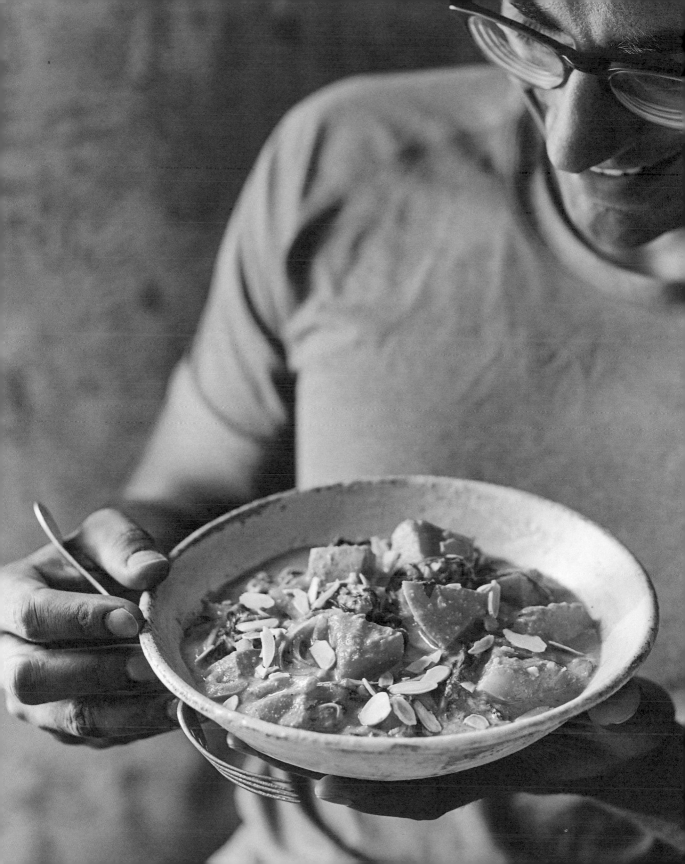

The pot does all the work in this recipe. All you need is the right combination of spices, condiments and herbs to give a stunning, authentic Caribbean flavour to simple beans.

Caribbean-style Black Bean Curry

1 Melt the coconut oil in a sauté pan over a low to medium heat, add the onion, ginger and garlic and fry gently for 2–3 minutes until softened.

2 Add the thyme, bay leaf, spices (including the Scotch bonnet chilli, if using), soy sauce and maple syrup, honey or sugar, and cook for a further minute.

3 Add the beans, tomatoes and peppers and simmer for 10 minutes until slightly reduced and sticky.

4 Season to taste with salt and pepper and serve with a good squeeze of lime juice and the coriander leaves.

Cook's tips

If you find Scotch bonnet too fiery for your taste buds, just use a milder green or red chilli instead. Cook the curry for a bit longer to really bring out the incredible sweet, aromatic and chilli notes in this dish.

PREP 10 MINUTES/COOK 15 MINUTES

2 tbsp coconut oil
100g onion (about 1 small), finely chopped
20g piece of root ginger (about 2cm), grated
2 garlic cloves, grated
1 tsp dried or fresh thyme leaves
1 bay leaf
1 small cinnamon stick
1 tsp coriander seeds
¼ tsp ground allspice or 3 allspice berries
1 Scotch bonnet chilli (optional)
1 tbsp soy sauce
1 tbsp maple syrup, honey or brown sugar
400g tin black beans, drained and rinsed
400g tin chopped tomatoes
160g roasted red peppers from a jar, roughly chopped
sea salt and freshly ground black pepper

TO SERVE
juice of 1 lime
15g fresh coriander leaves, chopped

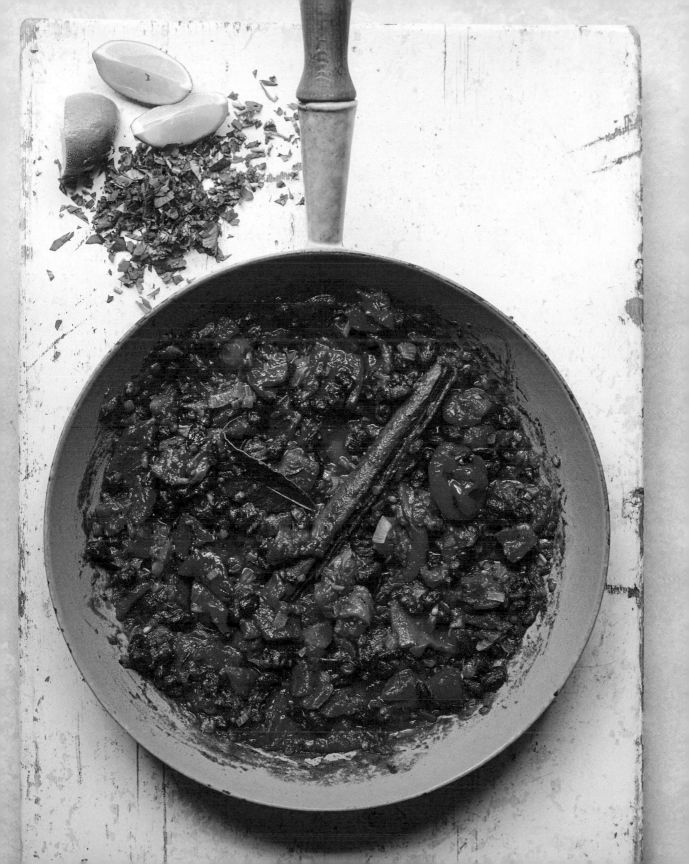

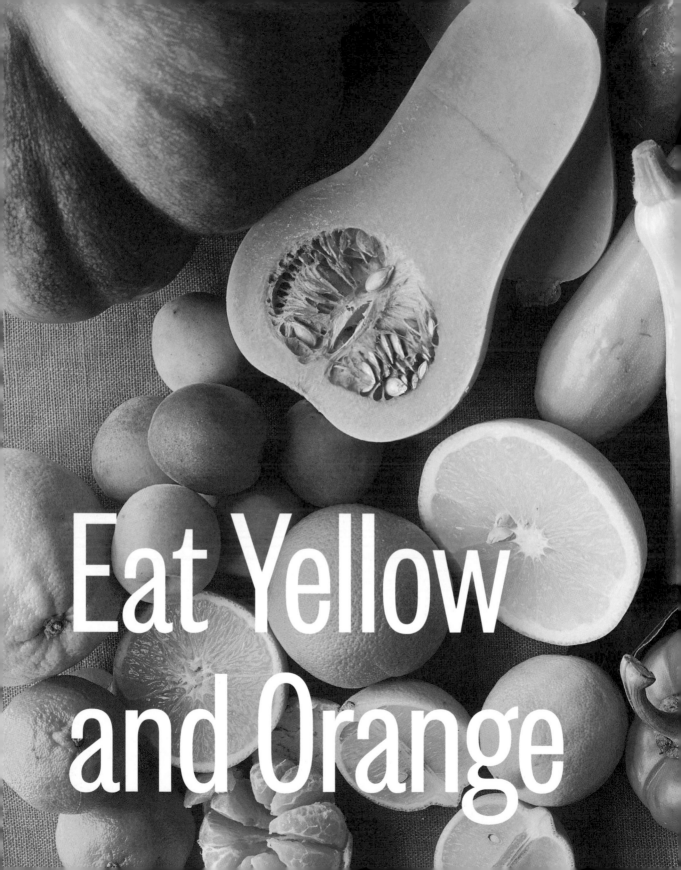

Eat Yellow and Orange

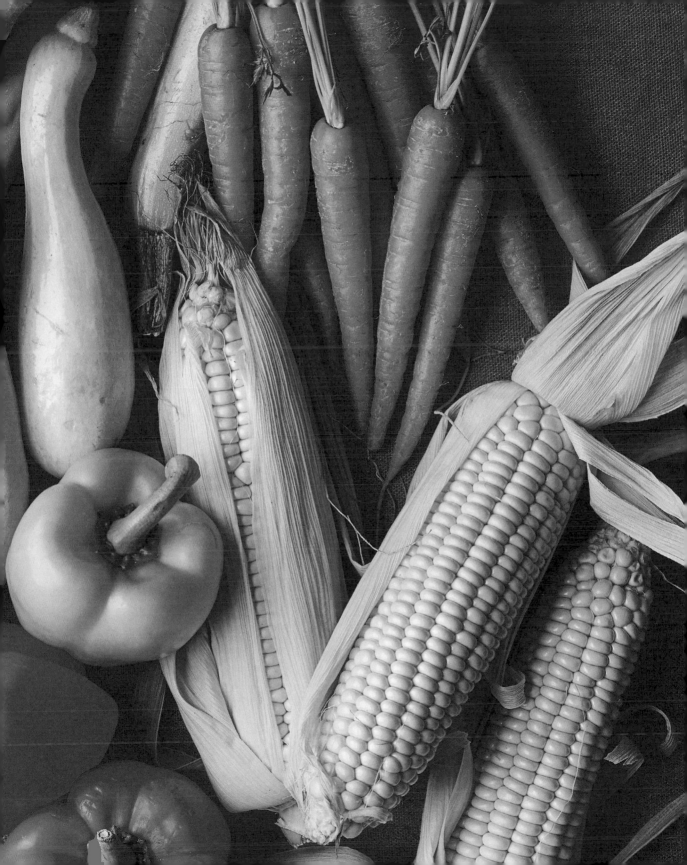

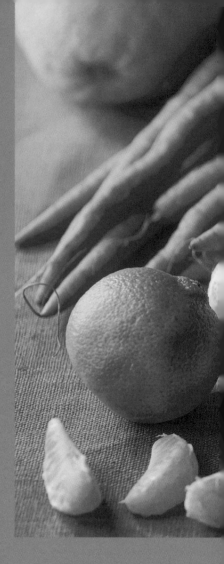

I tend to think of citrus fruits when I think of yellow ingredients, and their chemical constituents, such as limonene, carotenoids and the collection of flavonoids including naringenin, quercetin and apigenin (to name a few). These sharp-tasting fruits concentrate their chemicals in the rind and pith, which is why I tend to use the zest as well as the juice in dressings where possible.

Citrus as well as squash, courgettes and yellow peppers, can contribute to skin health by preventing extracellular matrix breakdown as well as providing good sources of vitamin C. These ingredients also contain precursors to vitamin A called beta-carotenes which, in combination with vitamin C and the plethora of other chemicals found in red and yellow ingredients, contribute to supporting our immune health.

When eaten, these types of chemicals, found in citrus, contribute to the overall antioxidant load of your diet, creating 'direct antioxidant' activity. In addition, they balance inflammation and have been shown in lab studies to change the expression of genes to lower inflammatory output. As well as inflammation lowering and immune supporting roles, these foods may be helpful in the prevention of cancers by limiting over-expression of inflammatory proteins and enhancing our organs' ability to expel environmental pollutants.

Corn is another great source of the carotenoids, called lutein and zeaxanthin, that have been shown in supplemental doses to help prevent cataracts and slow the progression of macular degeneration. Both fresh and frozen corn retain a lot of the nutrients locked inside, which is why my recipes can use either types and still provide a portion of your vegetable intake.

Carrots are widely known to contain large amounts of the precursors to

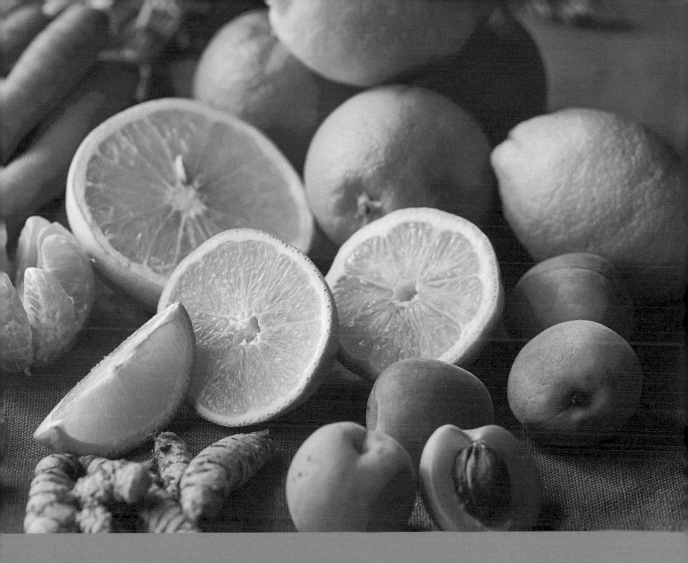

vitamin A. Owing to their phytochemical content and antioxidant capability, carrots and other yellow and orange vegetables are able to repair and prevent DNA damage in cells.

These foods contain an array of bioactives that may prevent arterial stiffening and aggregation of platelets that can lead to clotting, causing strokes and heart attacks. In addition to these chemicals, they also contain specialised fibres that can nurture your microbiota and maintain the structure and function of the digestive tract.

The reason why I highlight the importance of yellow and orange foods isn't to convince you to only eat these types of foods. It is to remind you of the relationship between the ingredients we put on our plate and their impact on our health. It's a reminder that to eat colourfully is to eat healthily, and explains why my dishes are formulated to provide as much variety as possible.

A generous amount of nut butter gives this curry a silky, voluptuous texture. It's brought to life with aromatic spices and sweet tomatoes.

Pumpkin Peanut Curry

1 Melt the coconut oil in a lidded deep sauté pan over a medium heat, add the pumpkin and cook for 5 minutes.

2 Stir in the garlic, ginger, whole chilli and the spices and cook for 2–3 minutes until fragrant.

3 Add the tomato purée and peanut butter, crumble in the stock cube and add the boiling water and chopped tomatoes. Season with salt and pepper and cook for another 5–6 minutes.

4 Add the spring greens. Cover and cook for another 5 minutes, until the greens are wilted.

5 Remove from the heat and serve with a good squeeze of lemon juice and the coriander and spring onion sprinkled over.

PREP 15 MINUTES/COOK 20 MINUTES

2 tbsp coconut oil

400g pumpkin (or squash), skin on, cut into 3cm cubes

1 garlic clove, thinly sliced

25g piece of root ginger (about 2.5cm), grated

1 red chilli (Scotch bonnet or long red chilli)

3 cardamom pods, cracked

1 tsp ground turmeric

1 tsp coriander seeds

1 cinnamon stick

1 bay leaf

2 tbsp tomato purée

100g smooth peanut butter

1 vegetable stock cube

450ml hot water

200g tomatoes, chopped

160g spring greens, chopped

sea salt and freshly ground black pepper

TO SERVE

squeeze of lemon juice

20g fresh coriander, leaves and stalks finely chopped

30g spring onions (2–3), thinly sliced

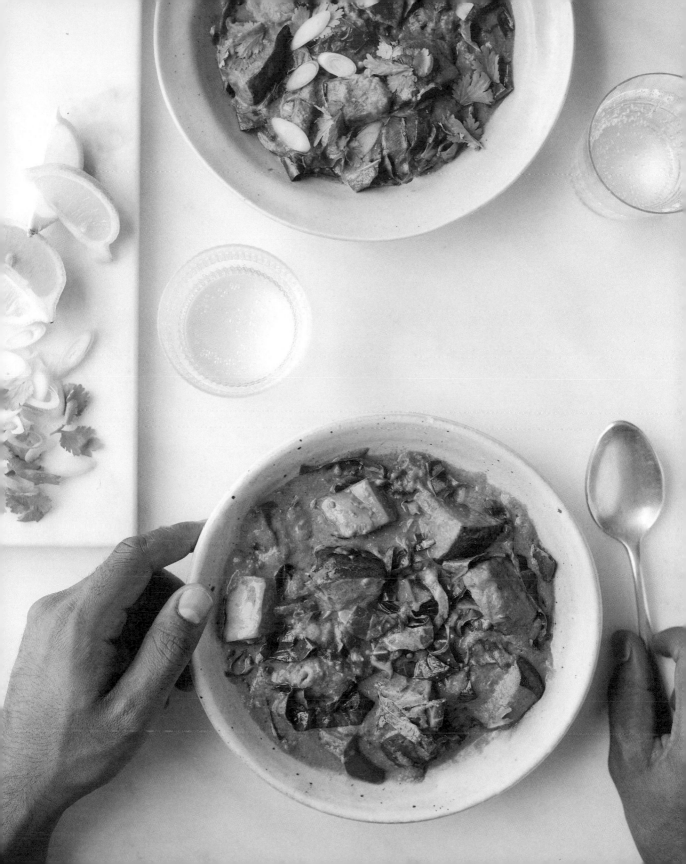

This is most definitely my favourite curry. Forgive the long list of spices (the dish is actually quite forgiving if you don't have them all) but the incredible blend of aromatics, almond flavour and bittersweet amchur is spectacular. You will thank me.

Almond Chicken Curry

1 Throw all the leaves and spices, ginger, garlic and almonds into a dry lidded pan and toast over a medium heat for 1–2 minutes.

2 Add the ghee or coconut oil and stir for another 1–2 minutes.

3 Add the chicken and stir to colour and coat in the spices for 2 minutes.

4 Add the water, tomato purée and tomatoes and season. Cover and simmer for 20 minutes until the chicken is cooked and the tomatoes have broken down to a thick sauce.

5 Add the spinach for the last few minutes of cooking until wilted.

6 Remove and serve scattered with the coriander and flaked almonds.

Cook's tip

Amchur powder has a sour, fruity flavour. If you can't get it, add 1 tablespoon tamarind paste with the tomatoes.

Variation

Use cooked chickpeas for a plant-based version.

PREP 15 MINUTES/COOK 30 MINUTES

12 fresh curry leaves
2 fresh kaffir lime leaves
½ tsp ground turmeric
1 tsp cumin seeds
1 tsp garam masala
1 star anise
½ cinnamon stick
3 cardamom pods, lightly crushed
1 tsp fenugreek seeds
1 tsp dried chilli flakes
2 tsp amchur (dried mango) powder
15g piece of root ginger (about 1.5cm), grated
3 garlic cloves, grated
60g ground almonds
1 tbsp ghee or coconut oil
200g skinless, boneless chicken thighs, sliced
400ml boiling water
2 tbsp tomato purée
250g ripe tomatoes, chopped
160g spinach, roughly chopped
sea salt and freshly ground black pepper

TO SERVE
15g fresh coriander leaves
1 tbsp flaked almonds

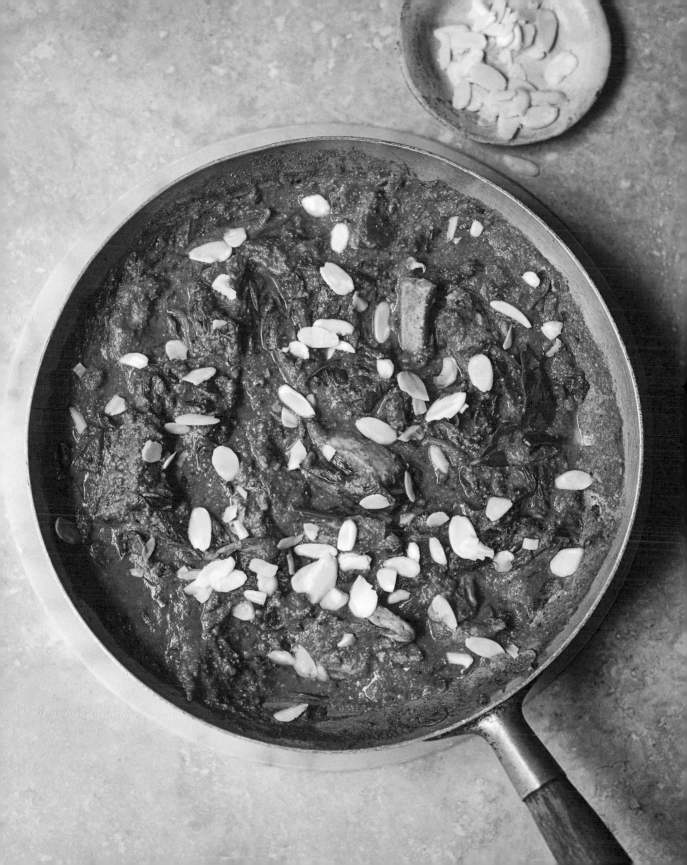

A classic yellow dhal is my go-to meal for a nutritious comforting hug at the end of a busy midweek day. The flavours work harmoniously together and cooking this is pure simplicity.

Coconut Yellow Dhal with Tamarind and Curry Leaves

1 Add the lentils to a deep saucepan with the coconut, tomatoes, curry leaves, lemongrass, tamarind paste and lime zest. Crumble in the stock cube and pour over the boiling water.

2 Simmer for 30–35 minutes until the lentils are tender, then season with salt and pepper.

3 Add the green beans, spinach and the extra 100ml water if needed, and cook for 5 minutes more.

4 Remove from the heat and stir in the coriander leaves. Top with red chilli and a squeeze of lime juice.

PREP 5 MINUTES/COOK 40 MINUTES

160g dried split yellow lentils, rinsed
60g desiccated coconut
250g tomatoes, roughly chopped
10 fresh curry leaves
1 stick of lemongrass, bruised
1 tbsp tamarind paste
finely grated zest and juice of 1 lime
1 vegetable stock cube
500ml boiling water (plus an extra 100ml if needed)
160g green beans, roughly chopped
50g spinach, roughly chopped
20g fresh coriander leaves
sea salt and freshly ground black pepper
1 red chilli, deseeded and finely chopped, to serve

Variation

Use frozen peas, sweetcorn or even chopped sugar snap peas instead of the green beans.

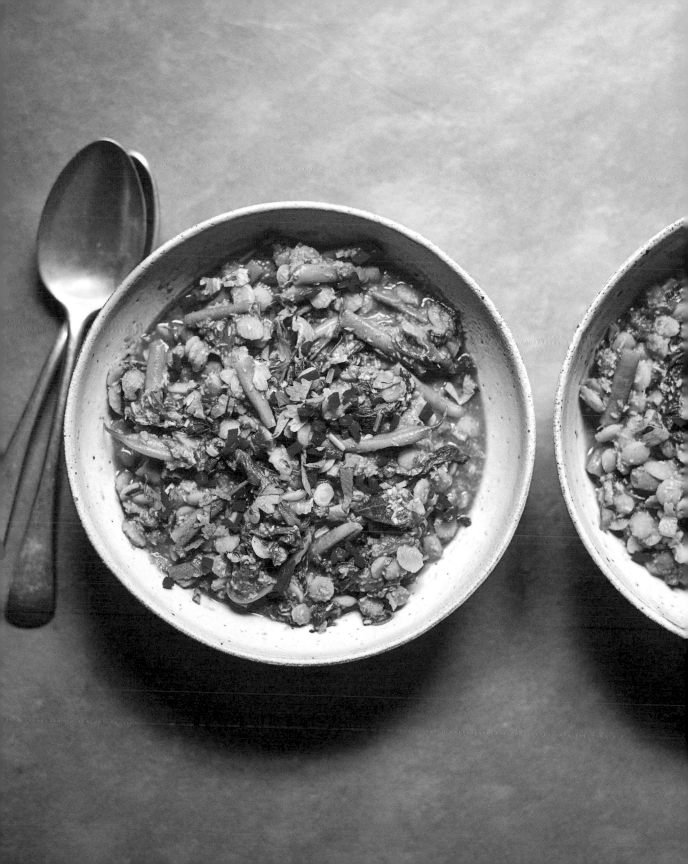

The flavour of mango pickle takes me back to my childhood growing up in an Indian household. It was a staple condiment on the dining table, just like salt and pepper. This beautiful ingredient is an incredible flavour powerhouse and this dish shows you how to make full use of it.

Mango Pickle and Squash Curry

1 Melt the oil or ghee in a sauté pan over a medium heat, add the squash and fry for 5 minutes until coloured on all sides.

2 Add the mango pickle and mustard seeds and cook for a minute more, until the seeds start to pop.

3 Quickly stir in the tomatoes, tomato purée and boiling water and season well with salt and pepper. Simmer for 15 minutes, until the squash is just tender.

4 Add the spinach and cook for a further 2–3 minutes. Remove from the heat and serve with a good scattering of toasted coconut flakes and chopped coriander.

PREP 5 MINUTES/COOK 25 MINUTES

2 tbsp coconut oil or ghee
300g skin-on butternut (or other) squash, cut into 1.5cm cubes
1 heaped tbsp mango pickle
2 tsp brown mustard seeds
400g tin chopped tomatoes
2 tbsp tomato purée
100ml boiling water
160g spinach, roughly chopped
sea salt and freshly ground black pepper

TO SERVE
30g toasted coconut flakes
15g fresh coriander leaves, chopped

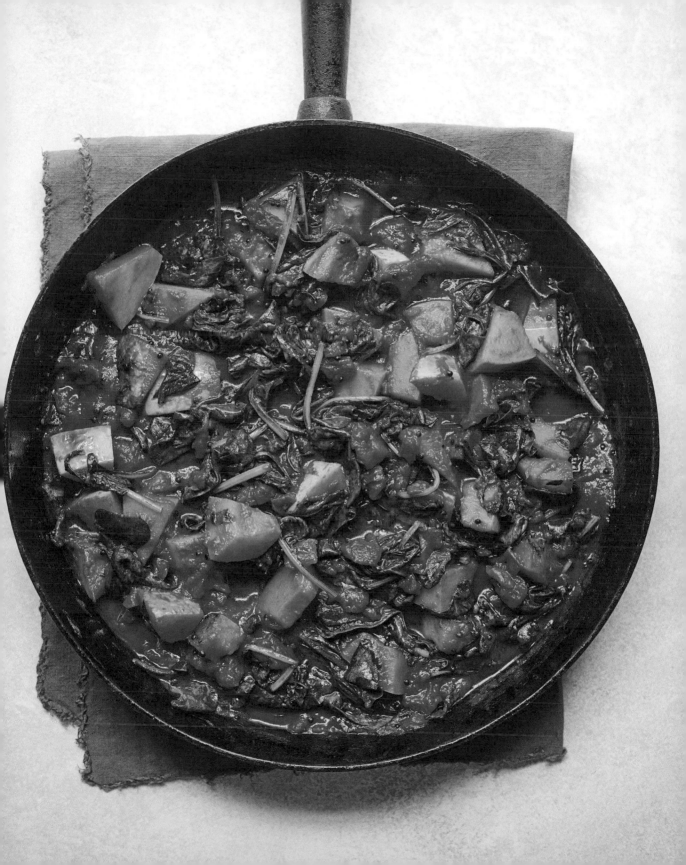

The sambal does all the work in this simple dish. The flavours beautifully complement each other and it is a joy to eat.

Sambal Red Lentils

1 Melt the coconut oil in a deep saucepan over a medium heat, add the onion, lemongrass, ginger and garlic and fry for 5 minutes, until softened.

2 Add the sambal paste, black pepper and lentils and fry for a further minute.

3 Stir in the coconut milk, boiling water, fish and soy sauces and simmer for 10–12 minutes until the lentils are tender.

4 Add the mangetout and peas and cook for a further 2–3 minutes.

5 Remove from the heat, season to taste and serve scattered with the coconut flakes and coriander.

PREP 5 MINUTES / COOK 20 MINUTES

1 tbsp coconut oil
100g red onion (about 1 small), finely chopped
1 stick of lemongrass, bashed
20g piece of root ginger (about 2cm), grated
2 garlic cloves, finely chopped
1 heaped tbsp sambal paste
½ tsp freshly ground black pepper
160g dried red lentils, rinsed
400g tin coconut milk
100ml boiling water
1 tbsp fish sauce
1½ tbsp soy sauce
160g sugar snap peas or mangetout, roughly chopped
160g peas (fresh or frozen)
sea salt

TO SERVE
20g coconut flakes (or dessicated coconut)
15g fresh coriander leaves, torn

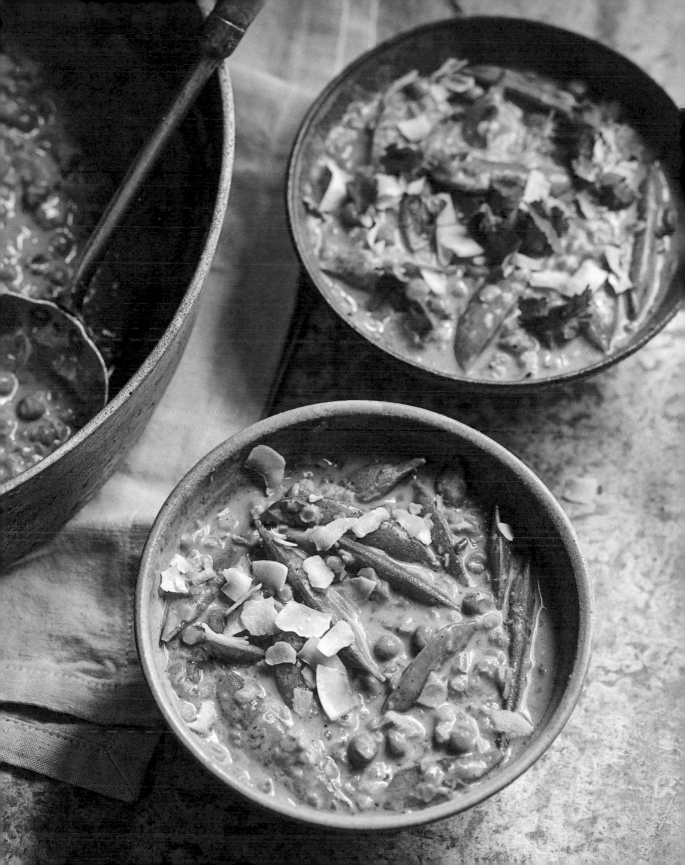

The gorgeous Caribbean flavours in this recipe work incredible magic on this simple collection of vegetables. Jackfruit is part of the breadfruit and fig family. When cooked, it has a meaty texture similar to pulled pork and it is widely used in vegan and vegetarian cooking.

Jerk-style Jackfruit and Sweet Potato Curry

1 Melt the oil in a sauté pan over a medium heat, add the onion and jackfruit and fry for 5 minutes.

2 Add all the spices, the sugar and herbs and cook for 2–3 minutes. Add the tomatoes, sweet potato, red pepper and crumble in the stock cube with the hot water.

3 Season with salt and pepper and simmer for 20 minutes until the sweet potato is tender.

4 Remove from the heat, add the lime juice and serve.

PREP 10 MINUTES/COOK 30 MINUTES

2 tbsp coconut oil

100g onion (about 1 small), roughly chopped

400g tin jackfruit, drained, rinsed and roughly chopped

1 tsp ground cumin

¼ tsp ground nutmeg

½ tsp ground allspice

1 tsp sweet smoked paprika

½ tsp ground cinnamon

pinch of cayenne pepper

2 tsp brown sugar

1 tsp fresh or dried thyme leaves

20g fresh flat-leaf parsley, leaves and stalks finely chopped

200g ripe tomatoes, roughly chopped

160g sweet potato, cut into 1.5cm cubes

160g deseeded red pepper (about 1 large), roughly chopped

½ vegetable stock cube

200ml boiling water

juice of 1 lime

sea salt and freshly ground black pepper

Kaffir lime, coconut and lemongrass is such a fabulous combination and here they completely transform simple split green peas into a balanced exotic dish.

Split Green Peas with Kaffir Lime and Coconut

1 Put the soaked and drained peas in a large sauté pan with the lime leaves, spices, lemongrass, coconut milk, boiling water and curry paste. Cover and simmer for 40 minutes until the peas are tender and falling apart. (Uncover for the last 10 minutes for a thicker consistency.)

2 When the lentils are cooked, season well, add the green beans and cook for a further 5 minutes.

3 Stir in the beansprouts and half of the coconut flakes and almonds.

4 Remove from the heat and serve scattered with the rest of the coconut and almonds.

PREP 5 MINUTES, PLUS SOAKING/
COOK 45 MINUTES

160g split green peas, soaked for 20 minutes in warm water

3–4 fresh kaffir lime leaves

1 cinnamon stick

2 cardamom pods, crushed

1 star anise

1 stick of lemongrass, bruised

400g tin coconut milk

200ml boiling water

1 tbsp Thai green curry paste

160g green beans, roughly chopped

160g beansprouts

20g coconut flakes

15g flaked almonds

sea salt and freshly ground black pepper

Cook's tip

You can use a tin or packet of ready-cooked lentils if you want to make the recipe quicker. Just use half the coconut milk and water and reduce the simmering time by half.

Tempeh is a fermented soybean product packed with protein, dietary fibre and vitamins. It originates from Indonesia and has a dense and chewy texture, as opposed to tofu's silky smooth texture. I know tempeh isn't everyone's favourite ingredient but trust me, it's because you haven't experienced it at its best. The flavours in this dish are phenomenal and the texture of tempeh suits this method of cooking.

Tempeh Red Curry

1 Melt half the coconut oil in a large casserole dish over a medium heat, add the tempeh and fry for 3–4 minutes until browned all over.

2 Remove and set aside, then add the onions to the same dish with the rest of the oil and sauté for 3–4 minutes.

3 Add the curry paste and ginger and fry, stirring, for 2 minutes until coloured.

4 Add the mangetout, asparagus, peanut butter and coconut milk, season with salt and pepper and simmer for 7–8 minutes.

5 Return the cooked tempeh to the dish for the last 2 minutes of cooking.

6 Serve with the lime juice and garnish with the chopped coriander and peanuts.

PREP 10 MINUTES/COOK 20 MINUTES

2 tbsp coconut oil
200g tempeh (or firm tofu), broken into 2cm pieces
160g red onion (about 1 medium), thinly sliced
1 tbsp red curry paste (or any curry paste)
50g piece of root ginger (about 5cm), grated
160g mangetout or sugar snap peas
160g asparagus spears, roughly chopped
2 tbsp peanut butter (smooth or crunchy)
400g tin coconut milk
sea salt and freshly ground black pepper

TO SERVE
juice of 1 lime
20g fresh coriander, chopped
30g unsalted peanuts, chopped

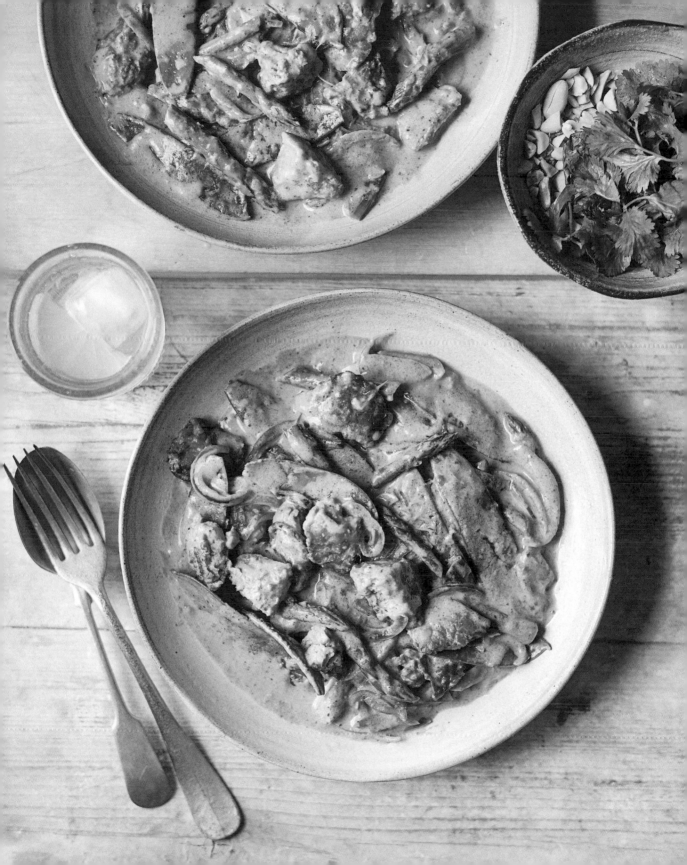

There is one lentil dish I find myself craving more than any other, and it's this dish. The umami blend of soy and fish sauces ripples through the sharp ginger and aromatics of cinnamon and star anise. This is a pleasure to cook and addictive to eat.

Malaysian-style Kari

1 Melt the coconut oil in a large saucepan over a medium heat, add the mustard seeds, cinnamon, star anise, shallots, curry leaves (if using), garlic and ginger and stir for 2–3 minutes until the oil and spices are fragrant.

2 Add the turmeric, soy sauce, fish sauce, aubergine and tomatoes, season and cook for a further 5 minutes before adding the lentils and stirring for another minute.

3 Add the boiling water and simmer for 35–40 minutes until the lentils are soft. Remove from the heat and either stick-blend or mash the mixture with a potato masher to create a lovely thick dhal.

4 Serve the dhal scattered with the coriander leaves.

PREP 10 MINUTES/COOK 45–50 MINUTES

2 tbsp coconut oil
1 tsp brown mustard seeds
1 cinnamon stick
1 star anise
120g shallots (about 2), finely chopped
8–10 curry leaves (optional)
2 garlic cloves, finely chopped
25g piece of root ginger (about 3cm), grated
1 tsp ground turmeric
1 tbsp soy sauce
1 tbsp fish sauce
160g aubergine (about 1 large), cut into 1.5cm chunks
200g ripe tomatoes, roughly chopped
200g dried split yellow lentils, rinsed
400ml boiling water
sea salt and freshly ground black pepper
10g fresh coriander leaves, to serve

Cook's tips

You can use cooked lentils from a tin – reduce the amount of boiling water by two-thirds and the cooking time (once the lentils are added to the aubergine, etc.) to 10 minutes.

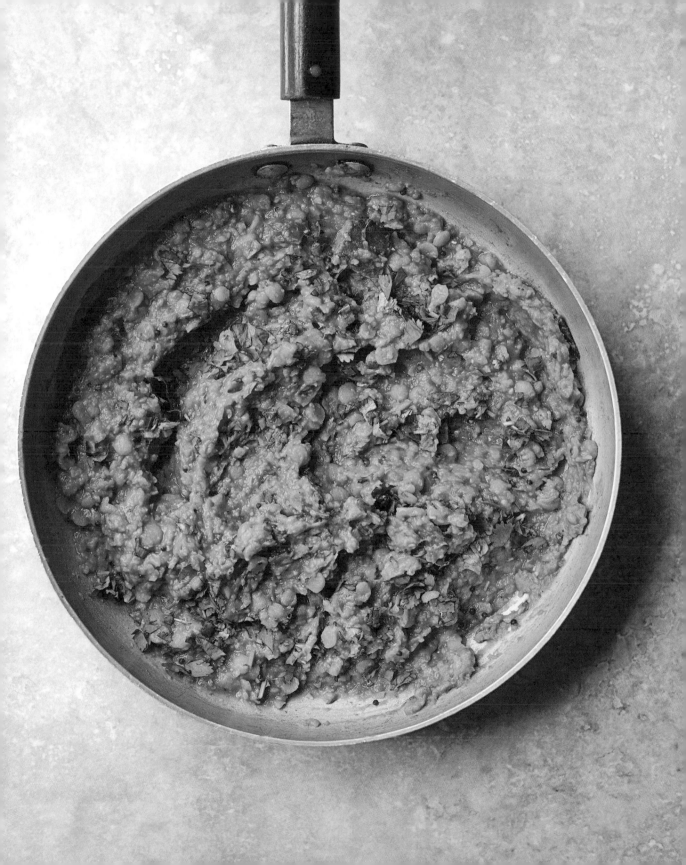

The addition of simple kitchen herbs is such an easy yet effective way of adding a delicious punch to simple lentils. This will transform your cooking!

Persian-style Brown Lentils with Mixed Green Herbs

1 Heat the oil in a shallow casserole dish over a low to medium heat, add the onion and fry gently for 5 minutes until softened.

2 Add the spices and cook for a further minute, then add the drained lentils and stir to allow the spices and lentils to mingle.

3 Add the passata, stock cube, water and honey or maple syrup. Stir in two-thirds of the herbs, cover and simmer for 30–35 minutes until the lentils are tender (add a splash of water if it starts to look dry). Season well when cooked.

4 Remove from the heat and serve scattered with the rest of the herbs, a drizzle of extra-virgin olive oil and a dollop of Greek yoghurt.

PREP 10 MINUTES/COOK 40 MINUTES

2 tbsp extra-virgin olive oil, plus extra for drizzling

160g onion (about 1 medium), diced

2 tsp sumac

1 tsp cumin seeds

1 tsp ground cinnamon

2 tsp sweet smoked paprika

160g brown lentils, rinsed and drained

160g passata

½ vegetable stock cube

200ml boiling water

1 tsp honey or maple syrup

25g fresh flat-leaf parsley, leaves and stalks chopped

25g fresh coriander leaves, chopped

20g fresh dill, chopped

sea salt and freshly ground black pepper

Greek yoghurt, to serve

Variation

Use sour cream or a plant-based yoghurt instead of Greek yoghurt, if you prefer.

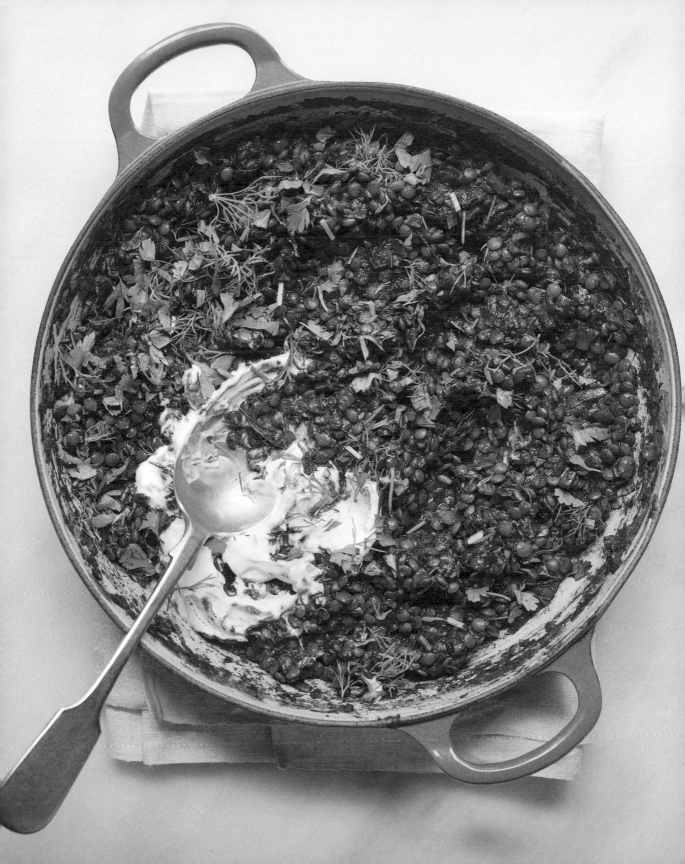

Casseroles and Stews

The flavour of Cajun spices and crab takes me back to my travels around Louisiana and the southern parts of North America. I love the combination and this stew is such an easy dish to cook and share with your family.

Cajun Crab Stew

1 Heat the oil in a casserole dish over a low to medium heat and add the onion, celery and parsley stalks, sautéing for 5 minutes.

2 Add the spices and fry for a further minute, then stir in the tomatoes and cook for 3 minutes until they start to break down.

3 Stir in the cornflour, then gradually add the boiling water, stirring, until smooth. Add the passata, kidney beans, crumble in the stock cube and a good amount of ground pepper and simmer for 10–12 minutes.

4 Fold in the crab meat for the last minute of cooking, season with black pepper and serve with a scattering of parsley leaves.

PREP 15 MINUTES/COOK 20 MINUTES

2 tbsp extra-virgin olive oil
160g onion (about 1 medium), finely diced
75g celery (1–2 stalks), chopped
20g fresh flat-leaf parsley, chopped stalks and leaves
1 tbsp Cajun spice mix
1 tsp fennel seeds
200g tomatoes, roughly chopped
2 tsp cornflour
200ml boiling water
200ml passata
400g tin red kidney beans, drained and rinsed
½ vegetable stock cube
200g white crab meat
sea salt

Cook's tip

You can use a Creole spice mix if you can't find Cajun spice mix, or a combination of cayenne pepper, fennel, dried oregano and smoked paprika in equal measures.

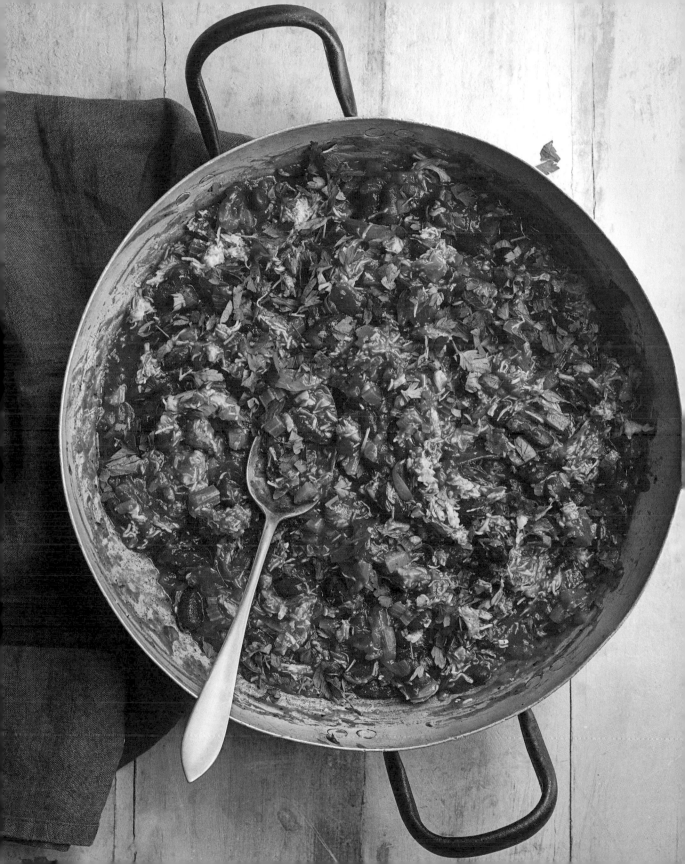

The holy trinity of celery, pepper and onion is the hallmark of Southern American cooking and this blend of vegetables with oregano and paprika is the epitome of comfort food. I adore this dish, with its hit of spice and indulgent chicken flavour.

Chicken Gumbo

1 Heat half the oil in a casserole dish over a high heat, add the chicken and cook for 4–5 minutes until brown all over. Remove and set aside on a plate.

2 Reduce to a medium heat and add the rest of the oil to the same casserole dish along with the celery, pepper, onions and garlic and fry for 5 minutes.

3 Add the paprika, oregano, cayenne pepper and tomato purée and season. Cook for 1 minute, then return the chicken to the dish.

4 Stir in the cornflour, crumble in the stock cube and add the water to the dish. Cover and simmer for 10–15 minutes until thickened.

5 Remove from the heat and serve the gumbo scattered with the dill.

PREP 15–20 MINUTES / COOK 25 MINUTES

2 tbsp extra-virgin olive oil

300–350g boneless, skinless chicken thighs (about 4), diced into 3cm chunks

160g celery (3–4 stalks), finely diced (reserve the leaves to garnish)

160g deseeded green pepper (about 1 large), finely diced

160g onion (about 1 medium), finely diced

2 garlic cloves, chopped

½ tsp smoked paprika

1 tsp dried oregano

generous pinch of cayenne pepper

1 tbsp tomato purée

1½ tbsp cornflour

1 vegetable stock cube

450ml boiling water

sea salt and freshly ground black pepper

15g fresh dill, chopped, to serve

Variation

If you want to make this veggie, swap the chicken for a tin of kidney beans and some chopped okra.

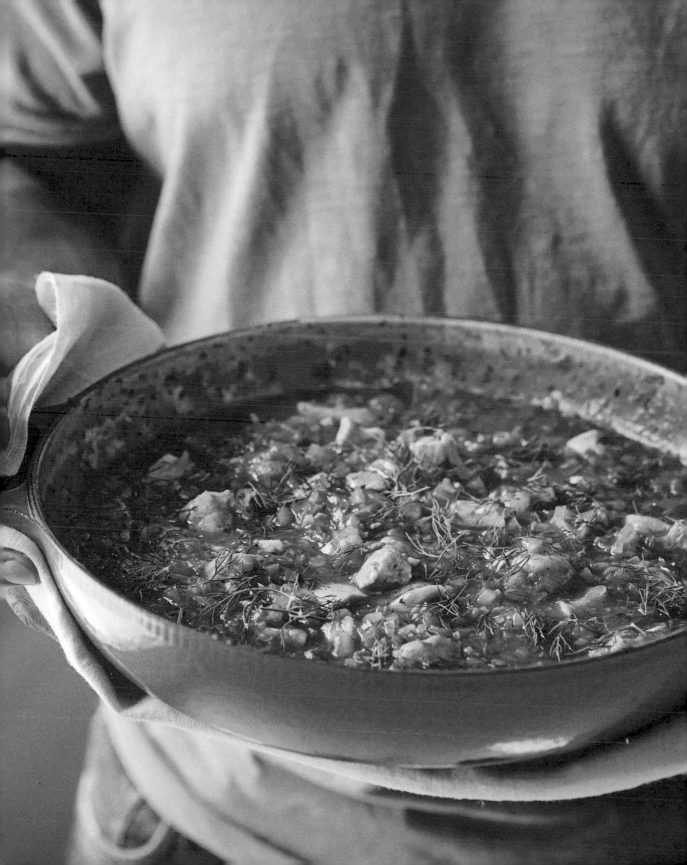

This dish takes me back to Guernsey, where I ordered this from a local beachside restaurant. Its indulgent, deep flavours are wonderful and perfect for sharing.

Prawn Bouillabaisse

1 Heat the oil in a shallow casserole dish over a low to medium heat, add the onions, fennel and leeks and cook gently for 10 minutes.

2 Add the garlic, paprika and chilli flakes and fry for a minute, then add the tomatoes and cook for 2–3 minutes more.

3 Crumble in the stock cube, then add the saffron, thyme leaves, bay leaf and water and simmer for 10 minutes.

4 Add the prawns and cook for another 2–3 minutes until they turn pink.

5 Remove from the heat and season to taste with salt and pepper. Serve scattered with parsley with lemon wedges and sourdough on the side.

Variation

You can easily make this plant-based by substituting the prawns for haricot beans or precooked puy lentils.

PREP 15 MINUTES/COOK 25 MINUTES

50ml extra-virgin olive oil
100g onion (about 1 small), finely chopped
160g fennel (about 1 small bulb), sliced
160g leeks (1 large or 2 small), roughly sliced
2 garlic cloves, grated
1 tsp smoked sweet paprika
½ tsp dried chilli flakes
200g ripe tomatoes, roughly chopped
1 vegetable or fish stock cube
pinch of saffron threads
1 tsp fresh or dried thyme leaves
1 bay leaf
500ml boiling water
200g raw shelled king prawns, deveined
sea salt and freshly ground black pepper

TO SERVE
15g fresh flat-leaf parsley, chopped
lemon wedges
toasted sourdough bread

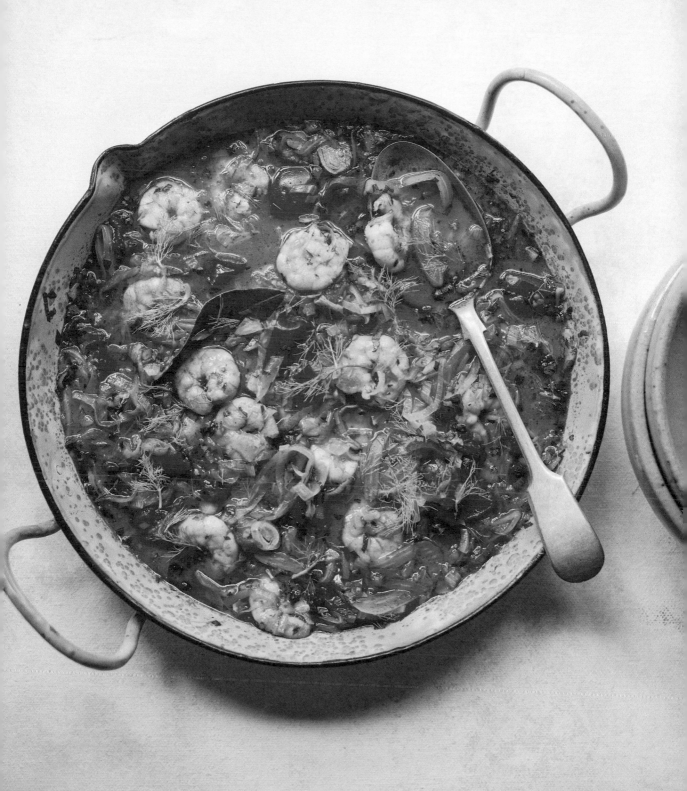

A veggie gumbo is just as satisfying as one made with seafood or chicken. The beautiful Creole flavours sing in complete harmony with the pepper and spring greens.

Green Gumbo

1 Heat the oil in a sauté pan over a low to medium heat, add the spring onion, celery, pepper and garlic and sauté gently for 5 minutes.

2 Add the Creole spice mix, cayenne pepper and crumble in the stock cube. Add the cornflour, tomato purée, butter and vinegar and stir for a minute.

3 Pour in the boiling water, bring to a simmer, add the greens and beans and cook for 5 minutes until the greens are tender and the sauce thickens and coats the vegetables.

4 Remove from the heat, season to taste with salt and pepper and serve with a scattering of parsley.

Variation

Try red kidney beans or even chickpeas as an alternative legume. Spinach and chard also work well instead of spring greens.

PREP 15 MINUTES/COOK 15 MINUTES

1 tbsp extra-virgin olive oil

100g spring onions (about 6), thinly sliced

75g celery (about 1½ stalks), chopped

160g deseeded green pepper (about 1 large), chopped

2 garlic cloves, thinly sliced

2 tsp Creole spice mix (or Cajun)

1 tsp cayenne pepper

1 vegetable stock cube

2 tsp cornflour

2 tsp tomato purée

2 tsp unsalted butter

2 tsp cider vinegar

400ml boiling water

160g spring greens, roughly chopped

400g tin black beans, drained and rinsed

sea salt and freshly ground black pepper

10g fresh flat-leaf parsley, leaves and stalks finely chopped, to serve

I find myself making variations of this brilliant autumnal hearty dish throughout the year. It's also a great way of using mustard, a condiment I sometimes struggle to find inspiration for.

French Lentils with a Dijon and Red Wine Vinaigrette

1 Heat 1 tablespoon of the oil and the butter in a casserole dish or sauté pan over a medium heat, add the shallot and garlic and fry for about 2–3 minutes.

2 Add the carrots and leeks and fry for a further 5 minutes until softened.

3 Add the drained lentils and stock, and simmer for 20 minutes until the lentils are just cooked. Season with salt and pepper.

4 Meanwhile, mix the vinegar in a bowl with the mustard and seasoning, then whisk in the rest of the olive oil to make a dressing.

5 Remove the lentils from the heat, pour the dressing over the hot lentils, fold in the parsley and serve.

PREP 10 MINUTES/COOK 25–30 MINUTES

3 tbsp extra-virgin olive oil
15g unsalted butter
50g banana shallot (about ½), finely chopped
2 garlic cloves, grated
160g carrots (1 large or 2 small), finely diced
160g leeks (1 large or 2 small), thinly sliced
160g Puy lentils, rinsed and drained
1 vegetable stock cube dissolved in 400ml boiling water
1 tbsp red wine vinegar
2 tsp Dijon mustard
sea salt and freshly ground black pepper
20g fresh flat-leaf parsley, finely chopped, to serve

This recipe is a gorgeous use of mixed mushrooms and sage: a flavour combination so well matched and that never disappoints.

Rice, Butter Bean and Wild Mushroom Stew

1 Heat the oil in a lidded casserole dish over a medium heat, add the onion, carrots and garlic and fry gently for 5 minutes until softened.

2 Add the mushrooms, increase the heat and fry for 2–3 minutes more, until they are coloured. Add the rice, chopped sage, soy sauce, stock cube and boiling water.

3 Stir the cashew butter into the mushroom mixture until combined. Season with salt and pepper, cover and simmer for 25 minutes.

4 Add the beans and cook for a further 10 minutes until the rice is cooked.

5 Remove from the heat and serve with extra pepper.

PREP 10 MINUTES/COOK 40–45 MINUTES

2 tbsp extra-virgin olive oil
100g onion (about 1 small), diced
160g carrots (1 large or 2 small), diced
2 garlic cloves, thinly sliced
160g mixed mushrooms and wild mushrooms (chestnut, chanterelle, morels etc.), torn if large
75g brown rice, rinsed
10g fresh sage leaves, chopped
1 tbsp soy sauce
½ vegetable stock cube
300ml boiling water
2 tbsp smooth cashew butter
400g tin butter beans, drained and rinsed
sea salt and freshly ground black pepper

Cook's tip

Fry a couple of sage leaves in another pan to garnish the dish if you're looking to enhance its visual appearance.

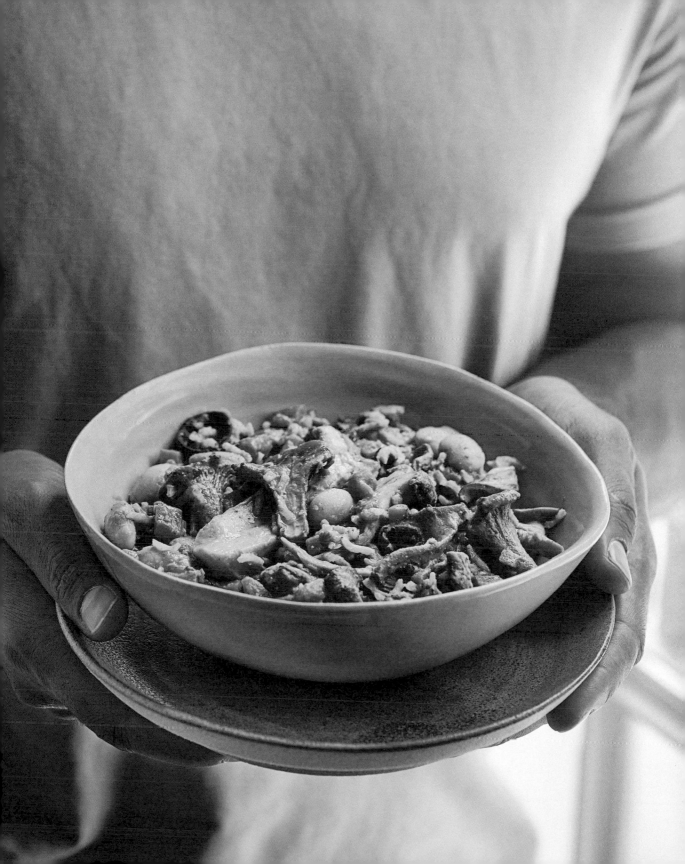

This hearty peasant dish works so well with the addition of sweet chestnuts and sage. It's a glorious combination that always hits the spot.

Tuscan Beans

1 Heat the oil in a lidded casserole dish over a medium heat, add the onion and carrot and fry gently for 5 minutes.

2 Add the garlic, butternut squash, bay leaf, sage and crumbled chestnuts and cook for a minute allowing the flavours to mingle.

3 Pour over the water, crumble in the stock cube and season with salt and pepper. Cover and simmer for 10 minutes until the squash is just tender.

4 Add the butter beans and cabbage leaves, re-cover and cook for a further 5 minutes, until the leaves are tender and the beans are warmed through.

5 Remove from the heat and serve scattered with the grated Parmesan and hazelnuts.

PREP 15 MINUTES / COOK 20 MINUTES

2 tbsp extra-virgin olive oil
120g onion (about 1 small), finely chopped
120g carrot (about 1 large), finely chopped
3 garlic cloves, grated
200g peeled and deseeded butternut squash, cut into 1cm cubes
1 bay leaf
6 fresh sage leaves
60g cooked and peeled chestnuts, crumbled
1 vegetable stock cube
300ml boiling water
400g tin butter beans, drained and rinsed
160g Savoy cabbage (about ¼ head), leaves separated and torn
sea salt and freshly ground black pepper

TO SERVE
2 tbsp grated Parmesan cheese
20g hazelnuts, chopped

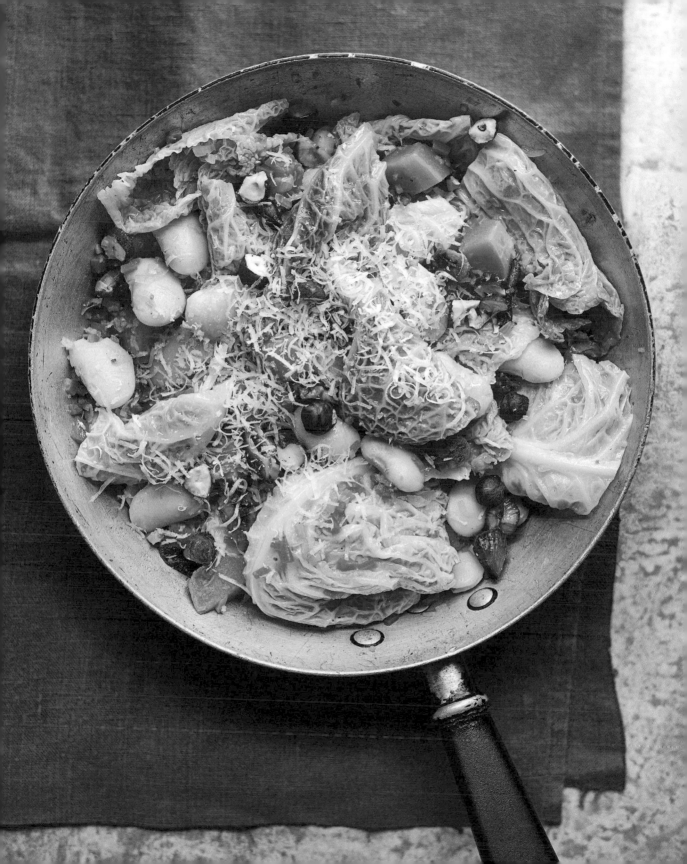

The combination of juniper berries, figs and walnuts is a fantastic blend, which works wonders in this simple dish. Trust me with the dried fruit here; it adds a wonderful complexity to the overall flavour.

Walnut and White Bean Stew

1 Heat the oil and butter in a casserole dish over a low to medium heat and add the onions, juniper berries, black pepper and thyme with a good pinch of sea salt. Sauté gently for 8–10 minutes until really softened.

2 Add the walnuts and dried figs, stirring for another 1–2 minutes to allow the flavours to combine.

3 Add the beans, stock and chard and simmer for 8–10 minutes until the chard is tender and the figs have softened.

4 Remove from the heat and serve with a scattering of parsley.

PREP 10 MINUTES / COOK 25 MINUTES

2 tbsp olive oil
1 tbsp unsalted butter
200g onion (about 1 large), finely chopped
6 juniper berries, bruised
1 tsp black peppercorns, coarsely crushed
5 sprigs of fresh thyme
100g walnut pieces, chopped
30g dried figs (about 2), finely chopped
400g tin white beans, drained and rinsed
300ml fresh chicken or vegetable stock
160g Swiss chard, finely shredded
sea salt
15g fresh flat-leaf parsley, chopped, to serve

Feta and honey is a delightful combination of salty and sweet that also adds a richness to this simple lentil and leek dish. In addition, rose harissa's gorgeous spicy perfume adds to the complexity of the stew's aromas.

Harissa Lentil Stew with Feta and Honey

1 Heat the oil in a casserole dish over a medium heat, add the leeks and sauté gently for 8–10 minutes until really soft.

2 Add the garlic and harissa paste and cook for a further minute, then stir in the lentils.

3 Add the tomatoes and boiling water and simmer for 22–25 minutes, until the lentils are tender but still have some bite. Season well.

4 Stir in the spinach and cook for a minute or two more, then remove from the heat.

5 Crumble over the feta, scatter with parsley and drizzle with the honey and a little more extra-virgin olive oil to serve.

PREP 10 MINUTES/COOK 35–40 MINUTES

2 tbsp extra-virgin olive oil, plus extra for drizzling
160g leeks (1 large or 2 small), roughly sliced
2 garlic cloves, grated
1 tbsp rose harissa or regular harissa paste
160g brown lentils, rinsed
400g tin chopped tomatoes
200ml boiling water
80g baby spinach, chopped
sea salt and freshly ground black pepper

TO SERVE
50g feta, crumbled
15g fresh flat-leaf parsley, leaves and stalks chopped
1 tbsp runny honey

Cook's tip

You can use tinned lentils, drained and rinsed, instead of dried – just halve the simmering time and use 100ml boiling water.

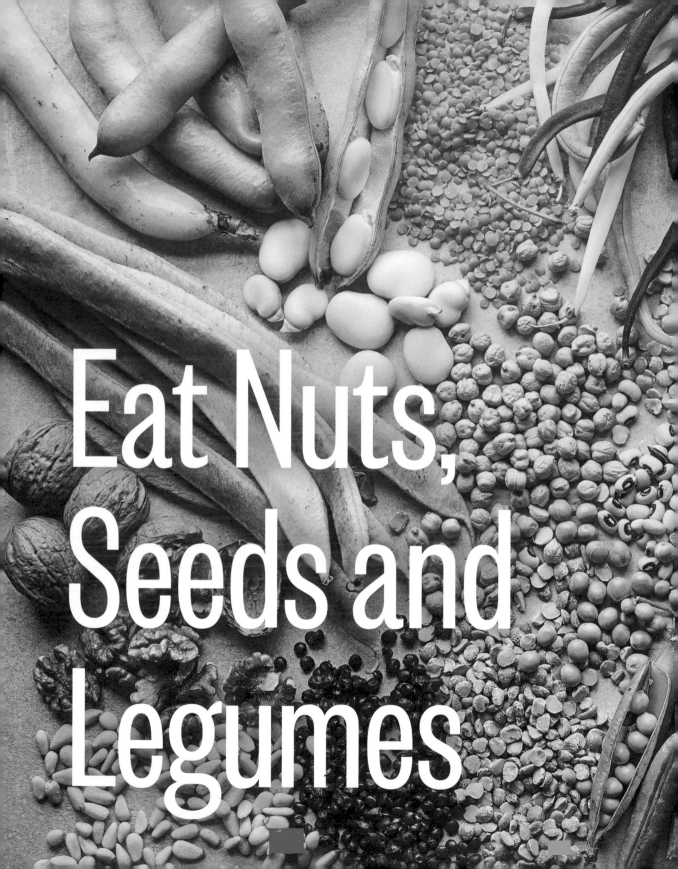

Eat Nuts, Seeds and Legumes

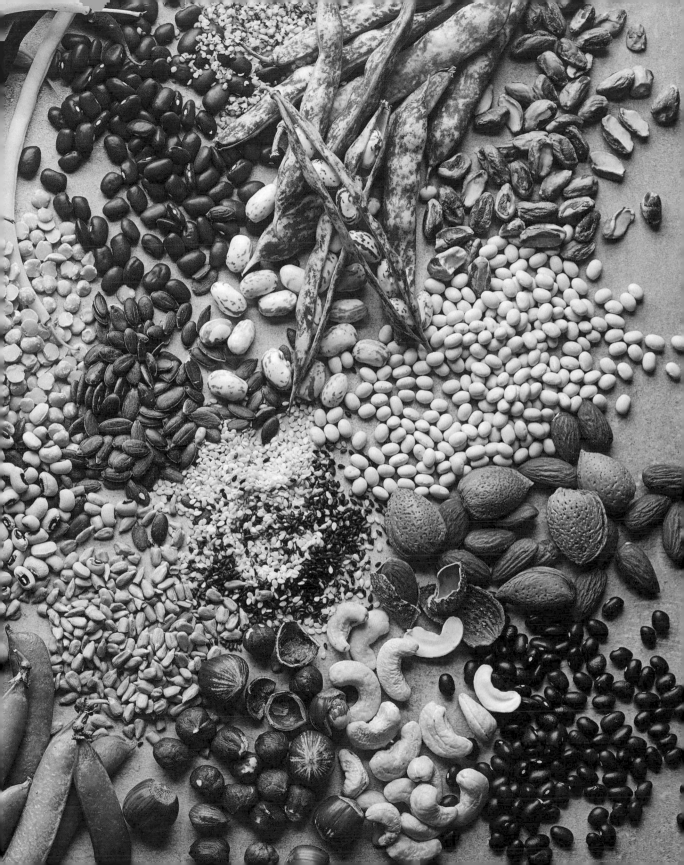

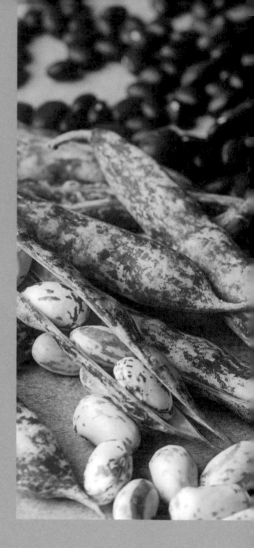

A high-fibre diet has been shown in many different studies to be associated with lower rates of cancer, heart disease and diabetes. Ingredients such as legumes, nuts and seeds are the easiest way to provide a number of different types of fibres that feed your gut microbiota and improve multiple aspects of health.

Most of my recipes try to utilise different types of pulses, beans and legumes such as chickpeas, broad beans, split peas, red lentils, black beans and more. These cheap, accessible sources of fibre and protein increase levels of beneficial microbes in the gut and the production of short-chain fatty acids that nourish your digestive tract and modulate inflammation.

I encourage eating different nuts and seeds as a snack, but I also incorporate a variety of them into recipes to provide texture, quality fats and flavour notes that blend well with the overall dish. Nuts and seeds are full of fibre as well as monounsaturated fats, vitamin E and short-chain omega 3 fatty acids that all contribute to protecting our heart and brain. A number of studies have demonstrated that higher consumption of these disease-fighting ingredients are associated with lower risks of high blood pressure and cognitive decline.

Studies that examine the potential protective mechanisms of these ingredients reveal that nuts and seeds also positively contribute to nurturing our gut microbes. Nut consumption is also related to longer telomere markers (the repeating bits of genetic material that protect our chromosomes) and better protection of our DNA that could improve health span as well as life span. The combination of micronutrients in your humble nut or seed includes vitamin E, zinc and magnesium, as well as phytonutrients such as gallic and ellagic acid that all contribute to less inflammation and improved cholesterol ratios, which lower cardiovascular risk.

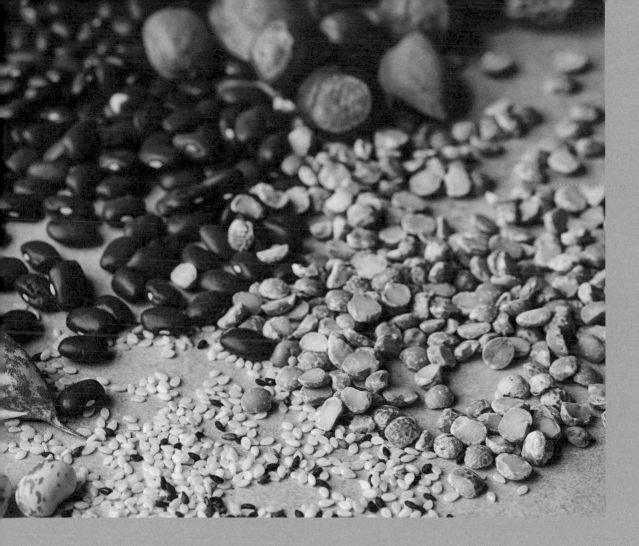

Cashew and sesame also contain bioactive, phenolic plant compounds called lignans, which are found in abundance in flaxseed, but also in legumes and other vegetables. When we eat these ingredients, the molecules are further digested by intestinal bacteria into unique compounds that exert oestrogenic effects. Flax, walnut, sesame and sunflower seeds are a few examples of ingredients that contain these phytoestrogenic plant compounds including isoflavones, lignans and coumestans. These are able to bind oestrogenic receptors and thus have oestrogenic activity in mammals. This sounds scary, especially in the wake of media articles that warn of the dangers of hormone disrupting foods, but it's these phytoestrogens that offer cardiovascular protection and can actually reduce the risk of high blood pressure, stroke and heart attacks. Analyses of these ingredients in foods tend to reveal positive results on health, rather than the opposite.

This meal may seem like a lunch or a main dish, but in Egypt and across the Middle East and Africa, it's breakfast! The sharp mint and citrus flavour works incredibly well with broad beans.

Ful Medames with Spinach and Garlic and Herb Dressing

1 Heat 1 tablespoon of the oil in a lidded sauté pan over a medium heat, add the cumin and coriander seeds and sauté for a minute.

2 Add the beans, tomatoes, spinach, sumac and boiling water. Season, cover and simmer for 14–15 minutes until the beans are soft.

3 Meanwhile, squeeze the juice of half a lemon over the red onion in a bowl, season and set aside.

4 In another bowl, mix the herbs, garlic, chilli (if using), the rest of the lemon juice and the remaining oil. Season and set aside.

5 When the beans are soft, mash in the pan lightly with a fork or potato masher. Spoon into a bowl to share, scatter with the onions, herb dressing and toasted pitta bread.

PREP 15 MINUTES/COOK 15 MINUTES

3 tbsp extra-virgin olive oil

1 tsp cumin seeds

1 tsp coriander seeds

400g tin fava beans or broad beans, drained and rinsed

200g ripe tomatoes, roughly chopped

160g spinach, finely chopped

1 tsp sumac

75ml boiling water

juice of 1 large lemon

50g red onion (about ½ onion), thinly sliced

10g fresh mint leaves, finely chopped

20g fresh flat-leaf parsley leaves, finely chopped

1 garlic clove, grated

1 long green chilli, finely chopped (optional)

sea salt and freshly ground black pepper

2 wholemeal pitta breads, toasted, to serve

Cook's tip

If you can get zhoug paste (a Yemenite paste), serve it with the beans, or add cinnamon.

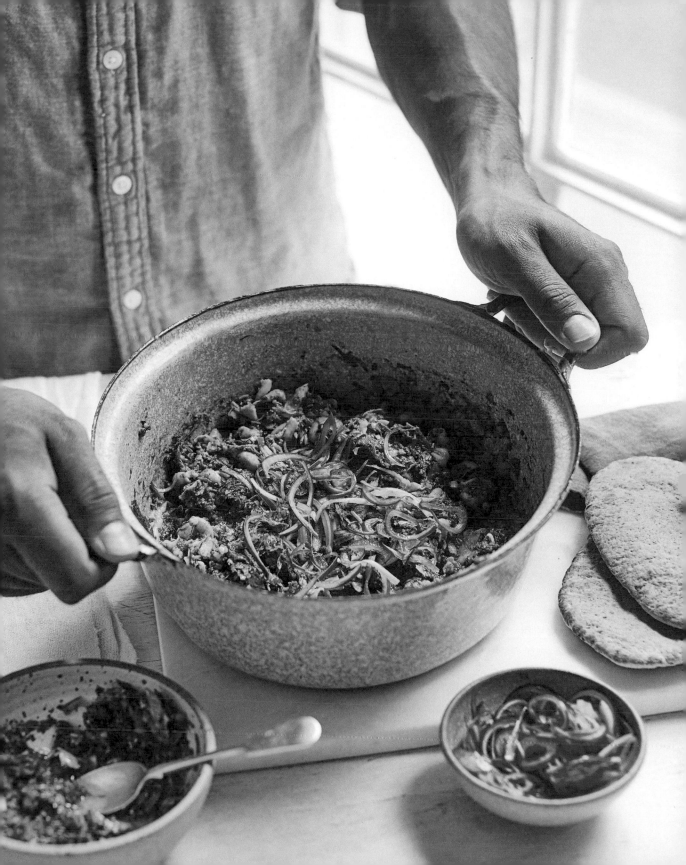

The delicious gochujang paste delivers an incredible sweet, tangy heat to this stew, and pairing it with black beans is an awesome way to deliver the flavour.

Korean-style Bean Stew

1 Heat the sesame oil in a casserole dish over a medium heat, add the spring onions, ginger and garlic and sauté gently for 5 minutes until softened.

2 Add the black beans, gochujang, cornflour and soy sauce and stir for a minute before adding the green beans, stock cube and boiling water.

3 Bring to a simmer, then add the tofu and cook for 5–6 minutes.

4 Remove from the heat and serve sprinkled with the sesame seeds and the rest of the spring onions.

PREP 10 MINUTES/COOK 15 MINUTES

2 tbsp sesame oil

160g spring onions (about 10), roughly sliced (reserving some for garnish)

50g piece of root ginger (about 5cm), grated

2 garlic cloves, grated

400g tin black beans, drained and rinsed

1 tbsp gochujang (or any chilli bean paste)

2 tsp cornflour

1 tbsp soy sauce

160g green beans, roughly chopped

½ vegetable stock cube

300ml boiling water

200g firm tofu (smoked flavour, or plain), cut into 1.5cm cubes

10g sesame seeds, to serve

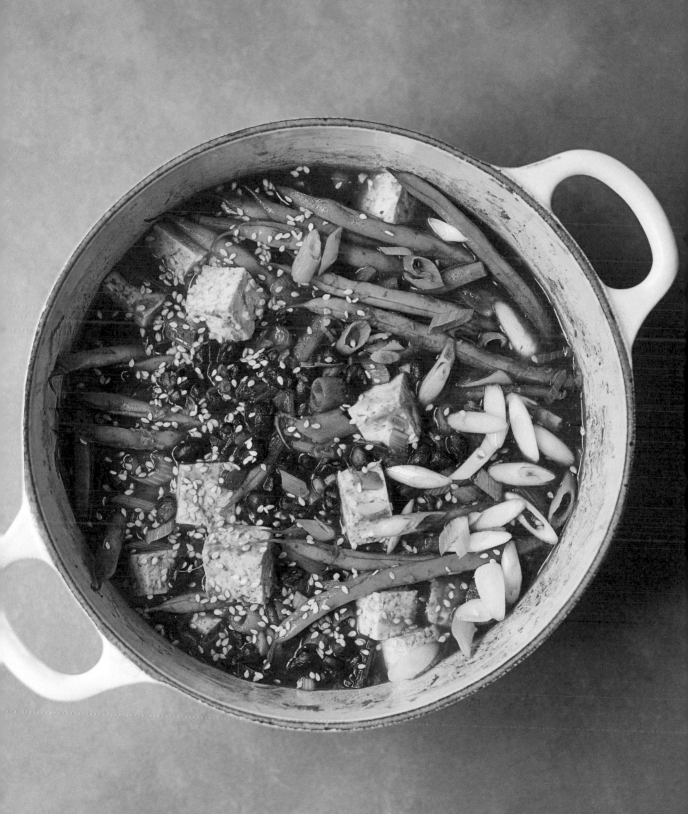

An indulgent Greek dish with punchy flavours, giouvetsi is usually made with stewing meat, but this vegetarian version has all the classic flavours without the heaviness. I love how easy the method is, too – just put everything in the casserole dish and let the oven do the work.

Red Bean Giouvetsi

1 Preheat the oven to 200°C/180°C fan/gas 6.

2 Put everything in a lidded casserole dish, except the feta and parsley. Season well and mix.

3 Cover with the lid, bring to a simmer on the hob, then transfer to the oven and cook for 20 minutes.

4 Remove from the oven and leave to stand for 5 minutes before removing the lid.

5 Remove the cinnamon stick and scatter with the feta and parsley to serve.

PREP 5 MINUTES/COOK 25 MINUTES

400g tin red kidney beans, drained and rinsed
400g tin chopped tomatoes
160g celery (3–4 stalks), finely chopped
1 bay leaf
1 cinnamon stick
2 tsp dried oregano
1 tsp ground cumin
1 tbsp balsamic vinegar
2 tbsp extra-virgin olive oil
60g orzo pasta
300ml boiling water
50g feta, crumbled
20g fresh flat-leaf parsley, leaves picked and chopped
sea salt and freshly ground black pepper

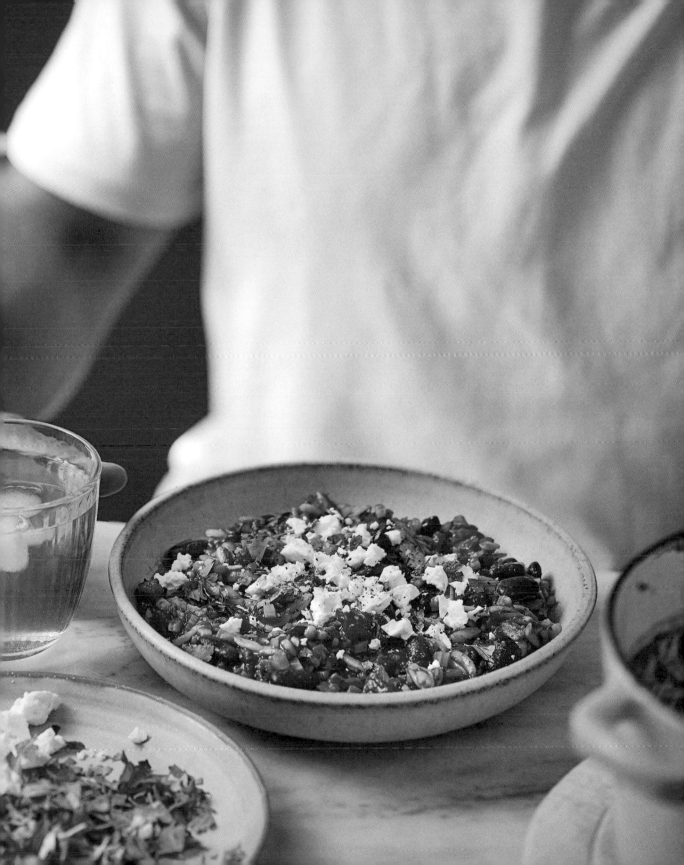

Soups and Broths

Bean soup and pesto is such a heart-warming comfort dish. This is something that I prepare for friends and family as a gesture of kindness and love. It's beautifully simple and generous.

Borlotti Bean Soup with Pesto

1 Heat the oil in a large saucepan over a medium heat, add the garlic, spices, parsley stalks and tomato purée, stir for 2 minutes.

2 Add the vinegar, beans, spring greens, cherry tomatoes, stock cube and boiling water. Cover and simmer for 15 minutes.

3 Meanwhile, make the pesto by finely chopping the basil, pine nuts and garlic together on a board, into a rough paste. Scrape into a bowl and add the cheese and oil.

4 Remove the soup from the heat, add most of the chopped parsley leaves, season to taste with salt and pepper and serve with a good dollop of pesto to stir in. Serve scattered with the rest of the parsley.

PREP 20 MINUTES / COOK 20 MINUTES

3 tbsp olive oil

4 garlic cloves, thinly sliced

2 tsp smoked paprika

1 tsp fennel seeds

25g fresh flat-leaf parsley, stalks and leaves chopped

2 tsp tomato purée

1 tbsp cider or red wine vinegar

400g tin borlotti beans, drained and rinsed

160g spring greens, shredded

400g tin cherry tomatoes

1 vegetable stock cube

650ml boiling water

sea salt and freshly ground black pepper

FOR THE QUICK CHOPPED PESTO

50g basil leaves

1 tbsp pine nuts

1 garlic clove, grated

15g grated Parmesan cheese

75ml extra-virgin olive oil

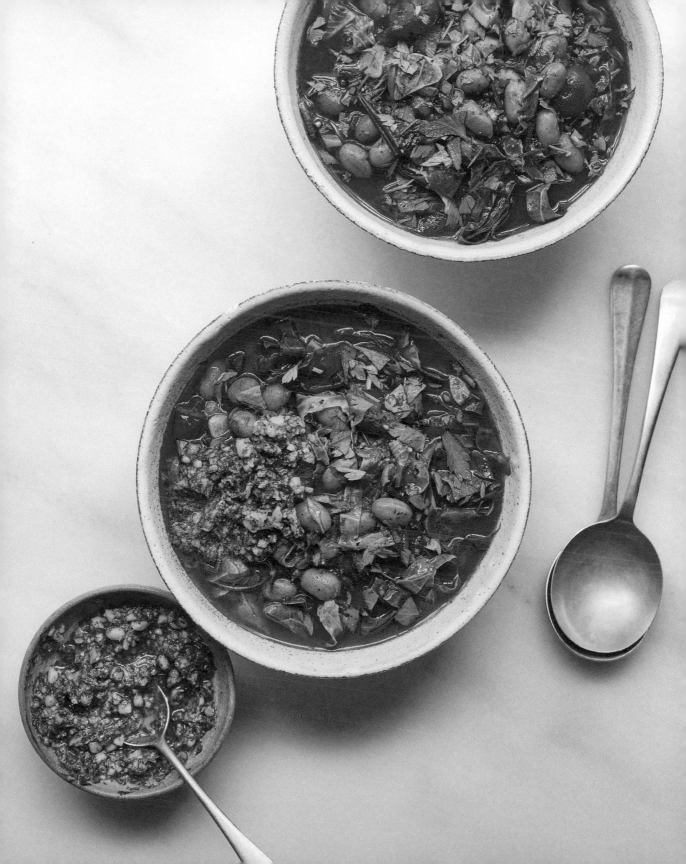

I have this dish when I need a quick health pick up. Packed full of vegetables, it's super delicious and uses beautiful sweet chestnuts to add an awesome texture.

5-a-day Bean Soup

1 Heat the oil in a high-sided saucepan over a medium heat, add the onion, celery and carrots and fry gently for 10 minutes until softened.

2 Add the garlic, beans, chestnuts and herbs and stir for a minute, then add the stock cube and boiling water. Season with salt and pepper, cover and simmer gently for 10 minutes, until the vegetables are really tender.

3 Remove from the heat, remove the bay leaf and blitz until smooth with a stick blender.

4 Serve with the Parmesan shavings, a drizzle of extra-virgin olive oil and some more black pepper.

PREP 15 MINUTES/COOK 20 MINUTES

3 tbsp extra-virgin olive oil, plus extra to serve
160g onion (about 1 medium), diced
160g celery (3–4 stalks), diced
160g carrots (1 large or 2 small), diced
2 garlic cloves, grated
400g tin cannellini beans, drained and rinsed
80g cooked and peeled chestnuts, crumbled
1 bay leaf
needles stripped from 2 rosemary sprigs
1 vegetable stock cube
500ml boiling water
sea salt and freshly ground black pepper
20g Parmesan cheese shavings, to serve

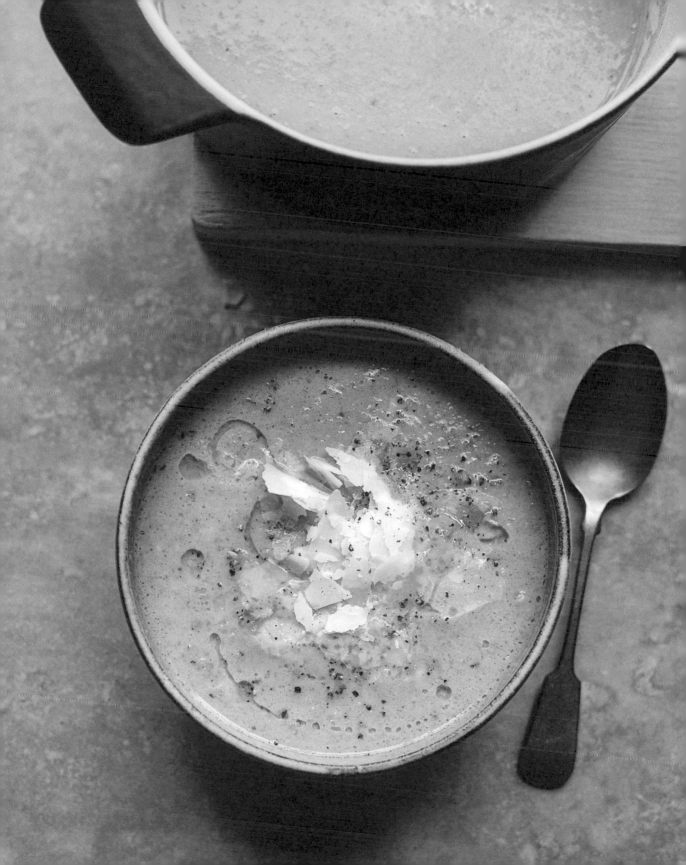

The olives add an amazing richness to this green soup, as well as a saltiness that pairs wonderfully with the sweet leeks.

 BEANS LEEKS

 SPINACH

Haricot Bean, Leek and Olive Soup

1 Heat the olive oil in a large saucepan over a medium heat, add the leeks and sauté for 5 minutes until softened.

2 Add most of the basil, and the rosemary, beans and olives, cooking for a further 5 minutes.

3 Add the stock cube, boiling water and spinach and simmer for 2–3 minutes until the beans are tender and the spinach wilted.

4 Remove from the heat and blitz until smooth with a stick blender.

5 Add lemon juice, salt and pepper to taste, then serve topped with the chopped hazelnuts, crumbled feta cheese, remaining basil leaves and a drizzle of oil.

PREP 10 MINUTES/COOK 15 MINUTES

3 tbsp extra-virgin olive oil, plus extra to serve
160g leeks (1 large or 2 small), roughly chopped
15g fresh basil, roughly chopped
10g fresh rosemary, needles stripped and finely chopped
400g tin haricot beans, drained and rinsed
50g pitted gordal or other large green olives
1 vegetable stock cube
750ml boiling water
160g spinach, roughly chopped
squeeze of lemon juice
sea salt and freshly ground black pepper

TO SERVE
40g hazelnuts, roughly chopped
40g feta cheese, crumbled

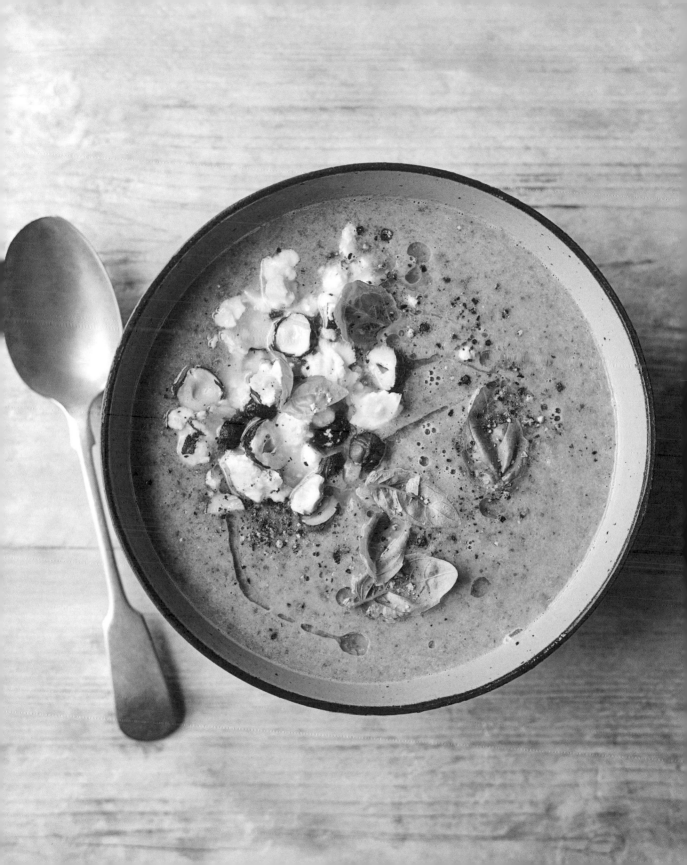

Most cauliflower soups use Mediterranean flavours, but this vegetable is a fantastic carrier of Indian flavours too, especially Indian masala, curry leaves and ginger.

Green Masala Cauliflower Soup

1 Melt the coconut oil in a saucepan over a medium heat, add the onions, ginger and chilli and fry gently for 5 minutes.

2 Add the dried spices, cauliflower florets and curry leaves and fry for 1–2 minutes to get some colour.

3 Add the stock cube and boiling water, season with salt and pepper, and simmer for 15 minutes.

4 Add the spinach and coconut cream and cook for 2 minutes more.

5 Remove from the heat, blend with a stick blender until smooth, and serve.

PREP 15 MINUTES/COOK 25 MINUTES

2 tbsp coconut oil

160g onion (about 1 medium), finely chopped

25g piece of root ginger (about 2.5cm), grated

1 long green chilli, deseeded and finely chopped

1 tsp fennel seeds

2 tsp brown mustard seeds

2 tsp mild curry powder

200g cauliflower (about ½ head), broken into florets

10–12 fresh curry leaves

1 vegetable stock cube

500ml boiling water

160g baby spinach

160ml tin coconut cream

sea salt and freshly ground black pepper

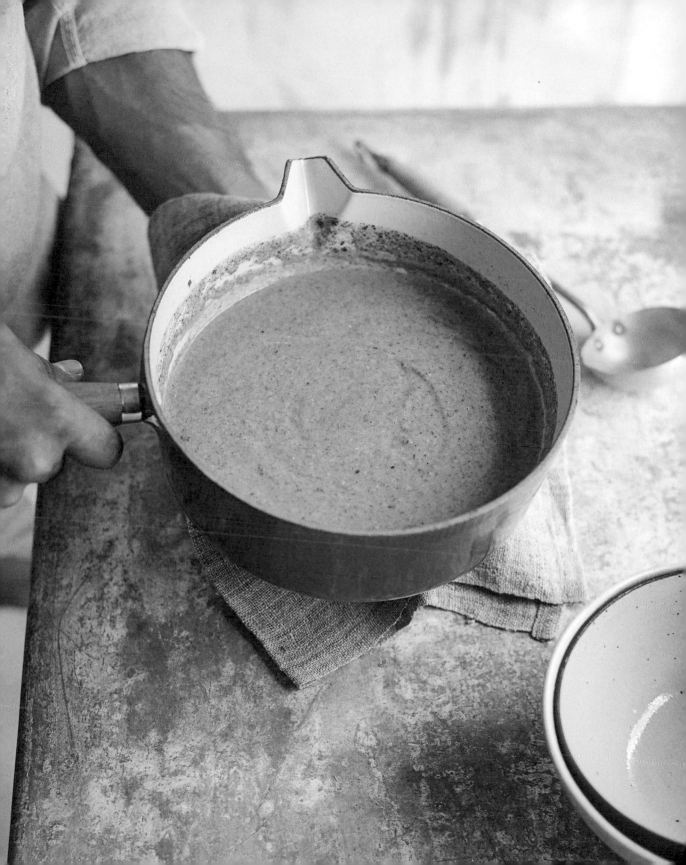

This tangy soup, punctuated with fresh chopped herbs, is such an unusual but delicious way to eat the humble chickpea.

Iranian-style Soup with Sumac and Fresh Green Herbs

1 Heat the oil in a large saucepan over a medium heat, add the onion and garlic and fry gently for 5 minutes.

2 Add the spices, chickpeas, half the dill and mint and the parsley stalks and cook for a minute more.

3 Stir in the spinach, stock cube and boiling water, season with salt and pepper and simmer for 5 minutes until all the vegetables are tender and the soup is fragrant.

4 Serve in bowls with a squeeze of lemon juice, a dollop of yoghurt, the remaining mint and dill, the parsley leaves scattered on top and a pinch of sumac.

Cook's tip

Try adding a teaspoon of harissa paste for an extra kick of spice.

PREP 10 MINUTES/COOK 10 MINUTES

2 tbsp olive oil

160g red onion (about 1 medium), thinly sliced

2 garlic cloves, grated

1 tsp sumac, plus extra for sprinkling

½ tsp ground turmeric

400g tin chickpeas, drained and rinsed

10g fresh dill, chopped

10g fresh mint leaves, chopped

10g fresh flat-leaf parsley, leaves and stalks chopped

160g baby spinach, roughly chopped

1 vegetable stock cube

500ml boiling water

sea salt and freshly ground black pepper

TO SERVE

lemon wedges

2 heaped tbsp Greek yoghurt (or plant-based alternative)

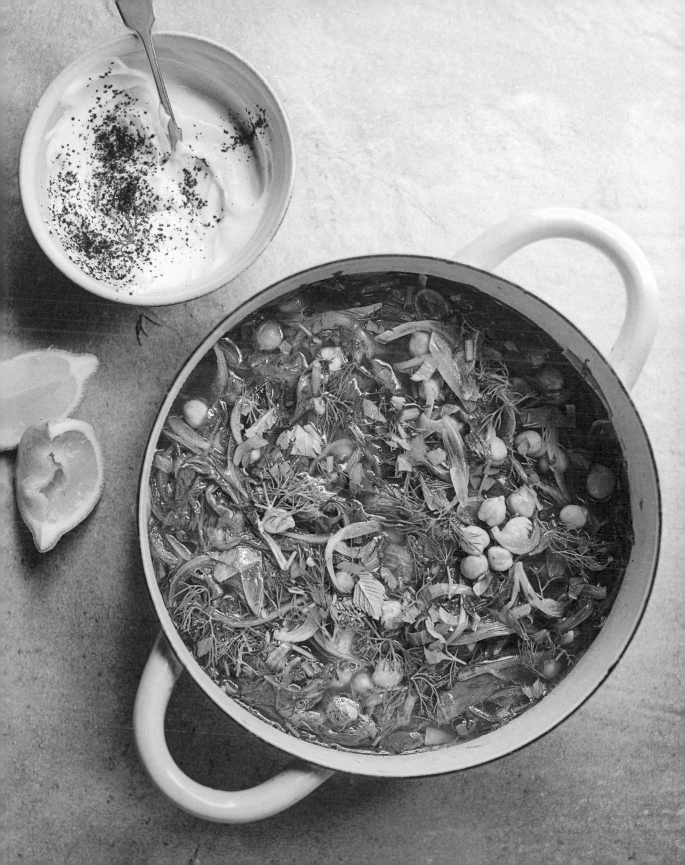

The rich, fiery blend of chipotle and black beans is complemented nicely here by the crunch of tortilla chips and mellow avocado, and the cumin, paprika and dried oregano carry the Southern flavour notes well.

Black Bean and Chipotle Soup

1 Heat the oil in a large saucepan over a medium heat, add the celery and garlic and fry gently for 5 minutes.

2 Add the paprika, cumin, oregano and black pepper and stir for a minute before tipping in the beans and adding the chipotle paste, stock cube and boiling water. Season with salt and pepper and simmer for 8–10 minutes.

3 Blend the mixture roughly with a stick blender (maintain some whole beans for texture).

4 Serve in bowls with sliced jalapeños, sour cream, coriander, crushed tortilla chips, avocado, lime juice and more black pepper, with a drizzle of extra-virgin olive oil.

Cook's tip

You can use any chilli paste if you can't find chipotle.

PREP 15 MINUTES/COOK 15 MINUTES

2 tbsp extra-virgin olive oil, plus extra for drizzling

160g celery (3–4 stalks), diced

2 garlic cloves, grated

1 tsp smoked paprika

2 tsp ground cumin

½ tsp dried oregano

good pinch of freshly ground black pepper

400g tin black beans, drained and rinsed

1 tbsp chipotle paste

½ vegetable stock cube

300ml boiling water

sea salt and freshly ground black pepper

TO SERVE

8 jalapeño slices from a jar

2 heaped tbsp sour cream or Greek yoghurt (or plant-based alternative)

15g fresh coriander leaves, roughly chopped

handful of blue corn (or other) tortilla chips, crushed

160g peeled and stoned avocado (1 large or 2 small), mashed

juice of 1 lime

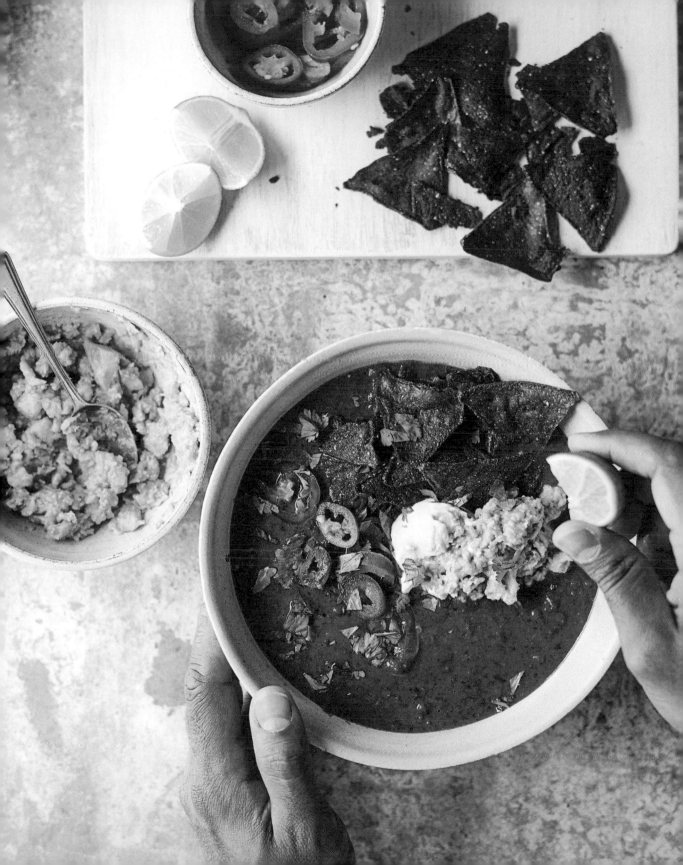

I use this broth as a way of kickstarting a healthy day, or when trying to recover from the inevitable viral illness. It's very simple, plus it delivers a delicious and pungent aroma of garlic and sage.

Ultimate Garlic Broth with Sage and Greens

1 Heat the oil in a large saucepan over a medium heat, add the garlic half, cut side down, and fry gently for 3–4 minutes until golden brown.

2 Add the boiling water to the pan along with the herbs, season with salt and pepper and cook very gently for 30–40 minutes until you have a deeply fragrant broth.

3 Add the celery and cook for about 5 minutes, then add the chard and spinach and cook for a further 5 minutes.

4 Add the rice noodles, remove from the heat and leave to stand for 5 minutes until the noodles are tender. Remove the garlic and serve.

PREP 10 MINUTES/COOK 1 HOUR

2 tbsp extra-virgin olive oil
1 whole garlic bulb, cut in half across the bulb
1 litre boiling water
15g fresh sage leaves
15g fresh flat-leaf parsley leaves
160g celery (3–4 stalks), roughly chopped
160g Swiss chard, roughly chopped
160g baby spinach, roughly chopped
100g vermicelli rice noodles, broken
sea salt and freshly ground black pepper

Cook's tip

Fry some extra sage leaves in butter until crispy, to garnish the broth.

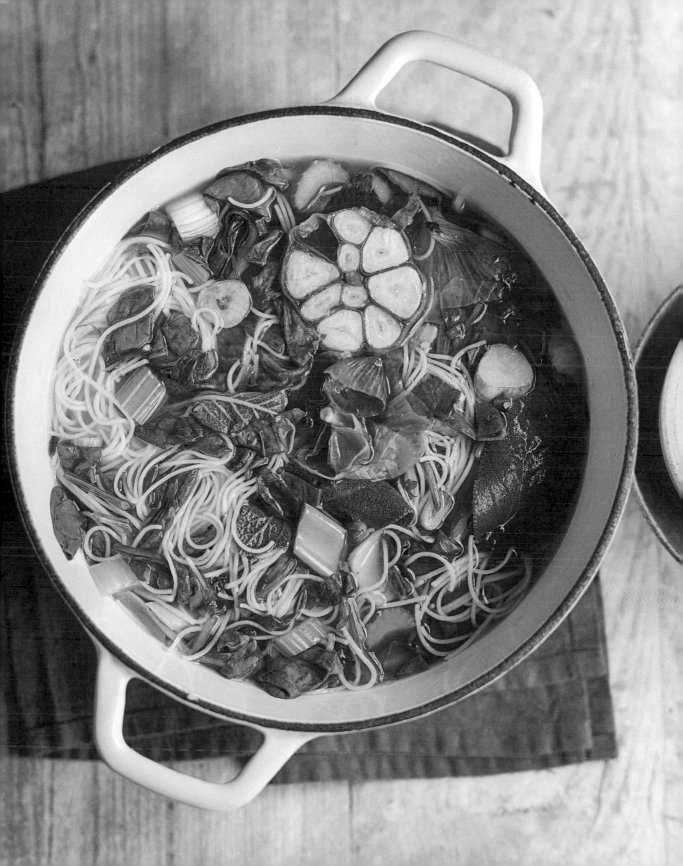

The flavours of kimchi and gochujang are so powerful, you barely need anything else to add flavour to this broth.

Korean-style Broth with Kimchi

1 Heat the oil in a saucepan over a medium heat, add the gochujang paste, garlic and spring onions and stir-fry for 2 minutes.

2 Add the stock and simmer for 5 minutes.

3 Add the kimchi and cabbage and simmer for another 10 minutes, until the cabbage leaves are slightly wilted.

4 Add the tofu to warm through. Remove from the heat, season to taste with salt and pepper and serve in deep bowls with a scattering of sesame seeds and some extra spring onions on top.

Cook's tip

You can also use brown miso paste instead of gochujang, with a dash of chilli powder.

PREP 5 MINUTES/COOK 15–20 MINUTES

1 tbsp sesame oil
2 tsp gochujang paste
4 garlic cloves, grated
160g spring onions (about 10), thinly sliced (reserve some for garnish)
600ml fresh chicken stock
160g kimchi
160g Chinese or Savoy cabbage, finely shredded
100g firm tofu, cut into 1cm cubes
sea salt and freshly ground black pepper
20g sesame seeds, to serve

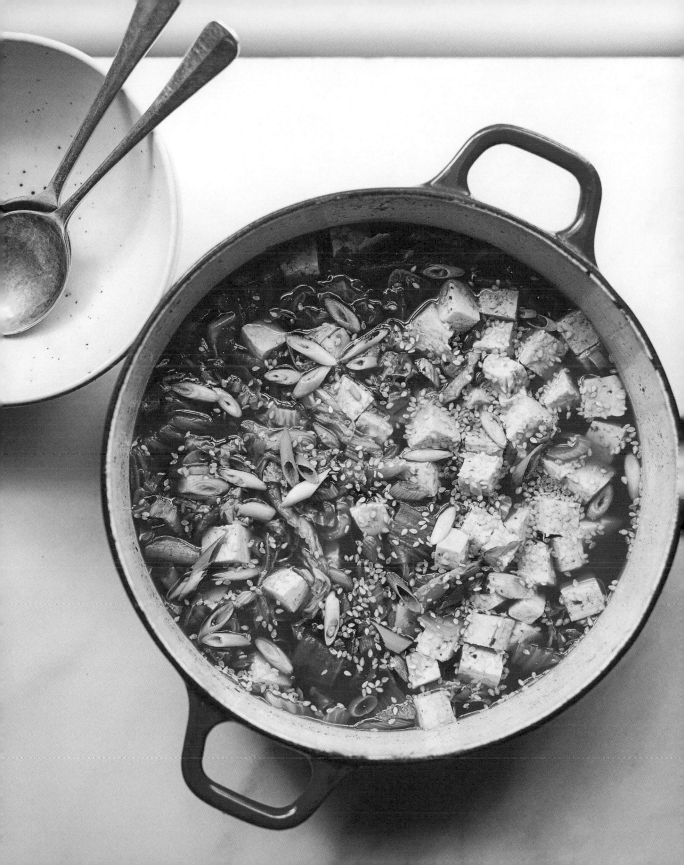

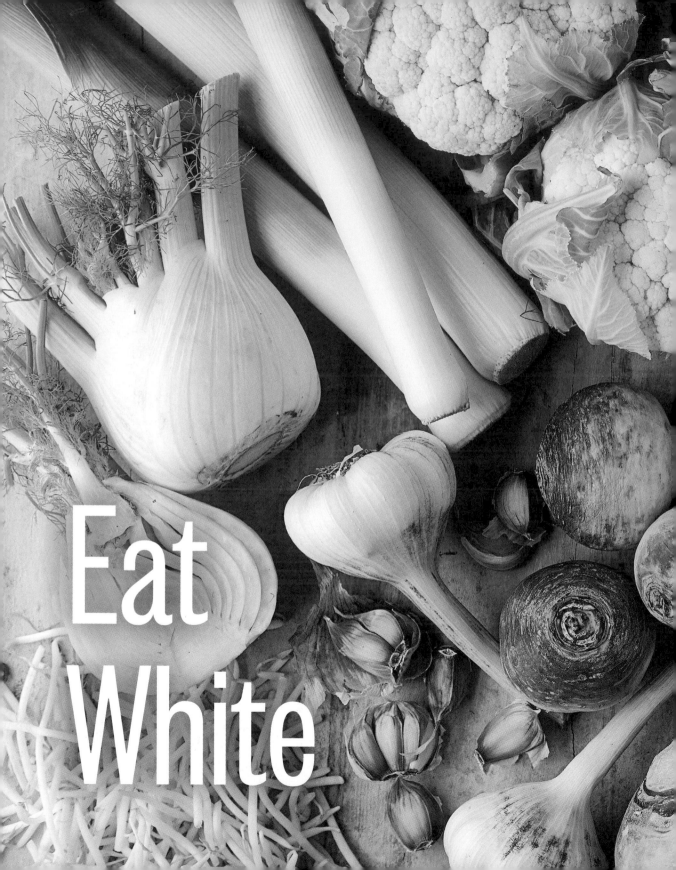

Eat
White

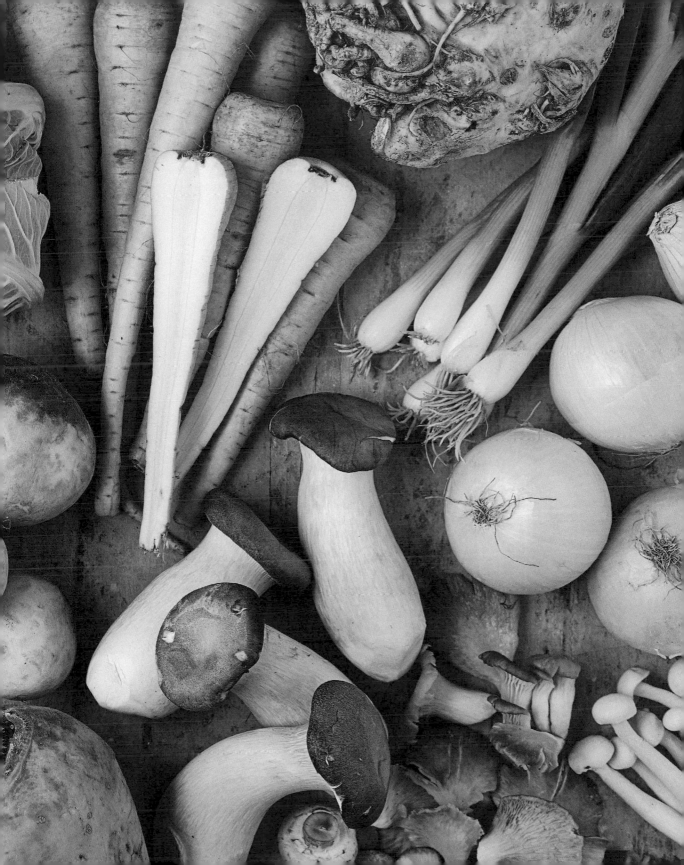

Considering all the beautiful colourful foods we have to choose from, we often forget about the humble 'white' foods that provide their own incredible array of benefits to our health. Mushrooms, swede and celeriac are all gorgeous examples of foods that we should certainly have on our plates, and my recipes contain a lot of them.

The inclusion of different types of mushrooms in a number of my recipes is because of their prebiotic fibre content that can potentially improve and enhance the function of your microbiota. In addition, these wonderful and accessible funghi contain bioactive compounds that can support your immune system and provide novel antioxidants that protect against oxidative stress and prevent oxidation of fats that can contribute to heart disease.

We don't often think of the nutritional value of garlic and onions, but they're wonderful additions to your diet. Pharmaceutical companies are looking to examine and extract chemicals from them that are recognised to have functional properties and they traditionally form the flavour base of dishes in a wide variety of cuisines including Indian, French and Chinese.

The phytochemicals, including flavonoids and sulphur amino acids, found in both red and white onions create a milieu of metabolites when digested by our bodies. These compounds, including thiosulphinates and sulphides, are thought to explain the anti-platelet activity of onions, which is why they may be beneficial for heart health. The only direct evidence we have of these benefits is from lab and animal model studies, but there is a promising correlation between onion consumption and heart health that needs further investigation.

Onions are also a source of the prebiotic fibre inulin, which we recognise as an important modulator of the gut microbe population that increases beneficial bifidobacteria and lactobacilli, which may improve the functioning of our immune system.

Celeriac has always had a reputation for being a 'medicinal' plant. The nutraceutical composition of celery (the shoots of the celeriac) reveals an abundance of plant chemicals most notably including apigenin, that serves multiple physiological functions, such as strong anti-inflammatory, antioxidant and antibacterial effects. Celeriac is also rich in fibre, minerals like calcium, phosphorus, iron, potassium and magnesium, vitamins like B1, B2, B3, A, C and flavonoids.

The humble swede, also known as rutabaga, is actually believed to be a brassica hybrid due to it being a cross between a turnip and a wild cabbage. Considering that brassicas are some of the most nutrient-dense vegetables you can get on the grocery shelves and the plant chemicals of them are known to have disease preventative properties, I made sure to include swede in some of my recipes to provide variety.

A number of interesting studies have examined rutabaga sprouts in the same way broccoli sprouts were investigated for antiproliferative properties (i.e. the ability to prevent cancer cells growing). Lab studies have demonstrated strong antioxidant and antiproliferative characteristics and this, plus the high fibre content, are reasons why we need to pay more attention to this simple vegetable and the many others on grocery shelves.

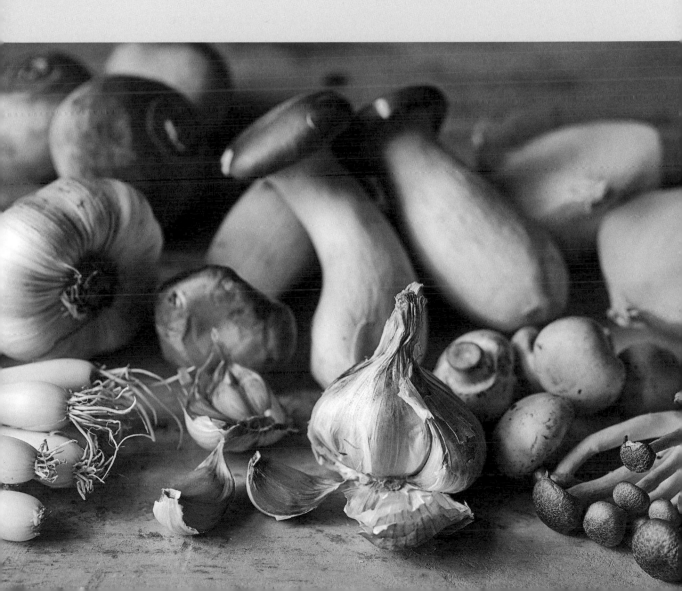

Italian brodo is typically made with chicken to make a delightful clear consommé, but fennel has such an aromatic and distinctive taste, it works really well as the primary flavour base. The orzo adds a bit of weight to the dish.

Fennel Brodo

1 Heat the oil in a saucepan over a low heat, add the fennel seeds and toast them for a minute until they smell fragrant.

2 Add the onion, garlic, chilli flakes, parsley stalks and fennel to the pan and cook for 5 minutes to soften.

3 Add the wine and let it bubble for a minute before adding the stock cube, boiling water and orzo. Season with salt and pepper and simmer for 6 minutes.

4 Add the broccoli and cook for a further 2–3 minutes, until the pasta and broccoli are tender.

5 Remove from the heat, stir in the parsley leaves and serve with lemon juice to taste and a scattering of Parmesan shavings.

PREP 10–15 MINUTES/COOK 15 MINUTES

2 tbsp extra-virgin olive oil
1 tsp fennel seeds
160g onion (about 1 medium), thinly sliced
1 garlic clove, thinly sliced
pinch of dried chilli flakes
20g fresh flat-leaf parsley, leaves picked and stalks chopped
160g fennel (about 1 small bulb), thinly sliced
100ml white wine
1 vegetable stock cube
800ml boiling water
50g orzo pasta
160g Tenderstem broccoli, roughly chopped
lemon juice, to taste
sea salt and freshly ground black pepper
20g Parmesan cheese shavings, to serve

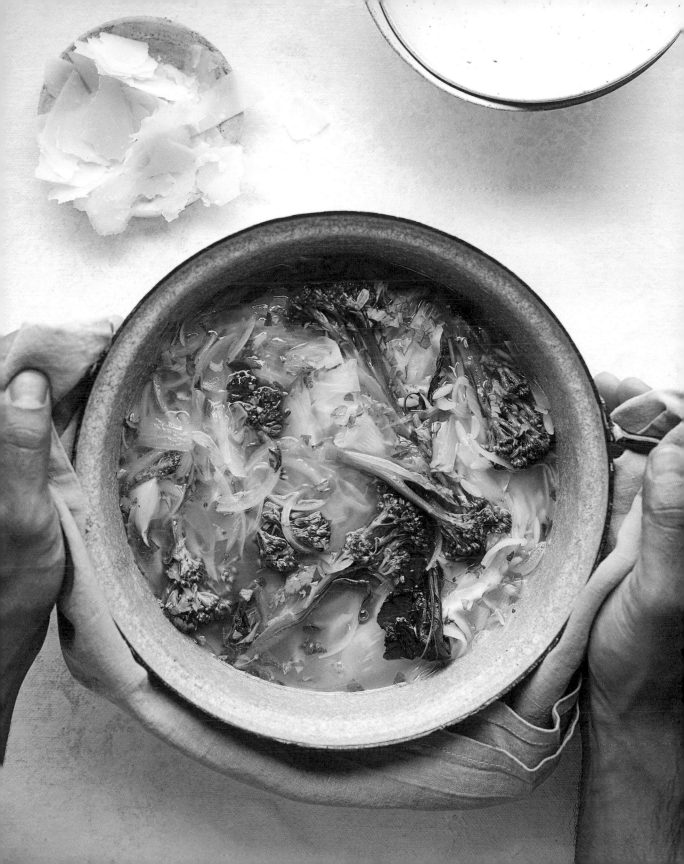

This is a brilliant way of injecting flavour into a classic ramen dish that would otherwise take hours to make: the combination of miso and dried mushrooms gives a great depth of flavour.

Chicken and Mushroom Ramen

1 Put the water, crumbled stock cubes, garlic, ginger, half the onions, the dried mushrooms and chicken in a large saucepan over a medium heat. Simmer for 10–12 minutes until the chicken is cooked through.

2 Remove the chicken from the pan, thinly slice and set aside.

3 Add the miso, mushrooms and spinach to the broth and cook for 2–3 minutes. Add the noodles, soy sauce and vinegar and cook for 1–2 minutes more until the noodles are tender.

4 Return the chicken to the pan with half the beansprouts. Serve with the remaining beansprouts, spring onions, chilli and sesame seeds.

PREP 10 MINUTES/COOK 15–20 MINUTES

800ml boiling water
2 chicken or vegetable stock cubes
1 garlic clove, thinly sliced
25g piece of root ginger (about 2.5cm), grated
75g spring onions (about 5), thinly sliced
10g dried wild mushrooms
150g boneless, skinless chicken thighs
1 tbsp brown or red miso paste
160g mixed exotic mushrooms such as shiitake, oyster and enoki, ripped
160g baby spinach leaves
120g ramen noodles
1 tbsp soy sauce
2 tsp rice vinegar
160g beansprouts

TO SERVE
1 red chilli, deseeded and thinly sliced
1 tbsp sesame seeds

Cook's tip

If the chicken has skin, remove, place on a baking tray, season and roast in a hot oven for 10–15 minutes until crisp. Crumble over the ramen to serve.

Variation

To make this gluten free, swap ramen for brown rice noodles and use gluten-free stock.

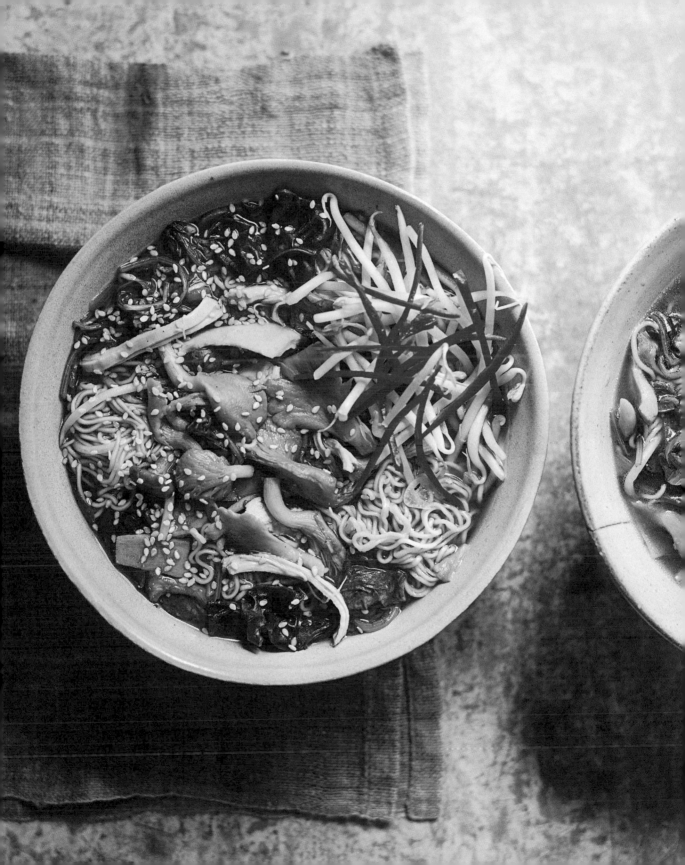

This dish is a delightful spring meal that uses the elements of the season and brings them together with an amazing pistou that is super-quick to make.

Asparagus, Courgette and White Bean Broth with Pistou

1 Add the stock cube and boiling water to a large saucepan with the horseradish and chilli and simmer for 5 minutes to allow the flavours to infuse the stock.

2 Add the courgettes and asparagus and cook for a further 1–2 minutes. Add the white beans and turn off the heat.

3 Meanwhile, make the pistou. Bash the garlic in a large pestle and mortar. Add the herbs, pine nuts and plenty of salt and pepper and grind to a coarse paste. Tip into a bowl and stir in the cheese and oil.

4 Season the broth to taste with salt and pepper (remove the whole chilli), then serve it topped with dollops of the pistou and some crusty bread.

PREP 10 MINUTES/COOK 10 MINUTES

1 vegetable stock cube
800ml boiling water
2 tsp fresh grated horseradish (optional)
1 red chilli, sliced lengthways
160g courgettes (1–2), finely diced
160g asparagus spears, sliced into 2cm pieces
400g tin white beans, drained and rinsed
sea salt and freshly ground black pepper
crusty bread, to serve

FOR THE PISTOU
2 garlic cloves, grated
15g fresh basil leaves, chopped
15g fresh flat-leaf parsley leaves, chopped
10g fresh mint leaves, chopped
1 tbsp pine nuts, finely chopped
1 tbsp grated Parmesan cheese
75ml extra-virgin olive oil

Cook's tip

If you can't get fresh horseradish, try using fresh ginger instead.

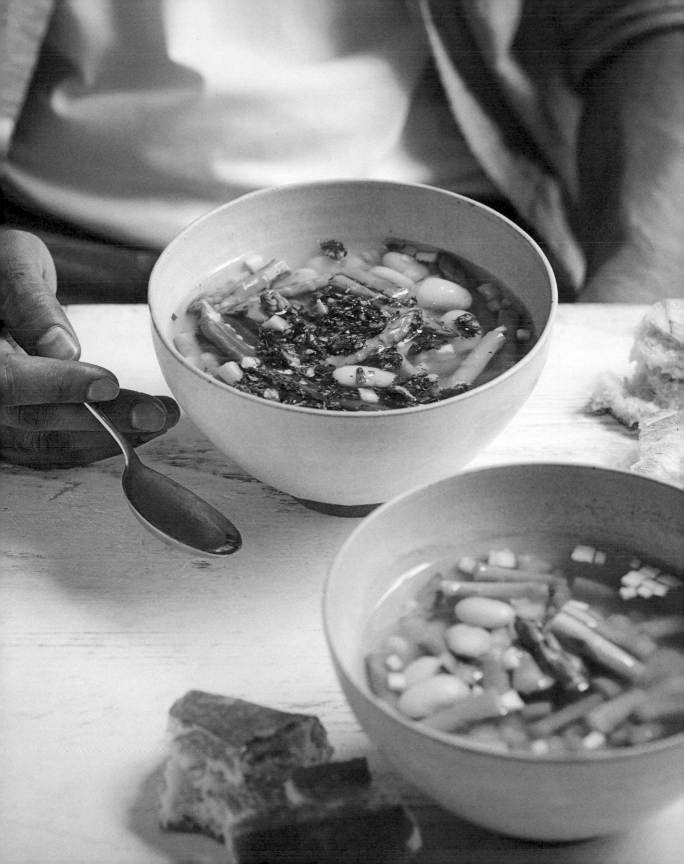

Stir Fries and Sautés

You may think the addition of tahini here is strange, but it combines so well with sugar, soy, vinegar and chilli that you won't make an Asian sauce again without it!

Sesame Rice Noodles with Carrots and Peas

1 Place the noodles in a bowl, cover with cold water and leave to stand for 10–15 minutes.

2 Drain the noodles, cook in boiling water for 2–3 minutes, drain, then rinse under warm running water. In a bowl, toss with 1 teaspoon of the sesame oil to stop them sticking.

3 Heat the remaining oil in a wok or large frying pan over a medium heat, fry the spring onions and garlic for 1 minute.

4 Add the tahini, vinegar, soy sauce, sugar, bean sauce and splash of water. Cook for 3–4 minutes, stirring, until you have a smooth sauce.

5 Add the cooked noodles and stir through the sauce until coated. Add the defrosted peas, carrots and coriander and cook, stirring, for a minute more.

6 Serve with sesame seeds, coriander, chilli and a squeeze of lime.

PREP 15 MINUTES/COOK 10 MINUTES

150g flat rice noodles
2 tbsp sesame oil
100g spring onions (about 6), sliced
2 garlic cloves, grated
60g dark (or regular) tahini paste
2 tbsp rice vinegar
2 tbsp dark soy sauce
2 tsp palm or light brown sugar
1 tbsp chilli bean sauce (optional)
160g frozen peas, defrosted
160g carrots (1 large or 2 small), coarsely grated or julienned
25g fresh coriander stalks and leaves, chopped, plus extra to serve

TO SERVE
10g sesame seeds, to garnish
1 red chilli, thinly sliced
juice of 1 lime

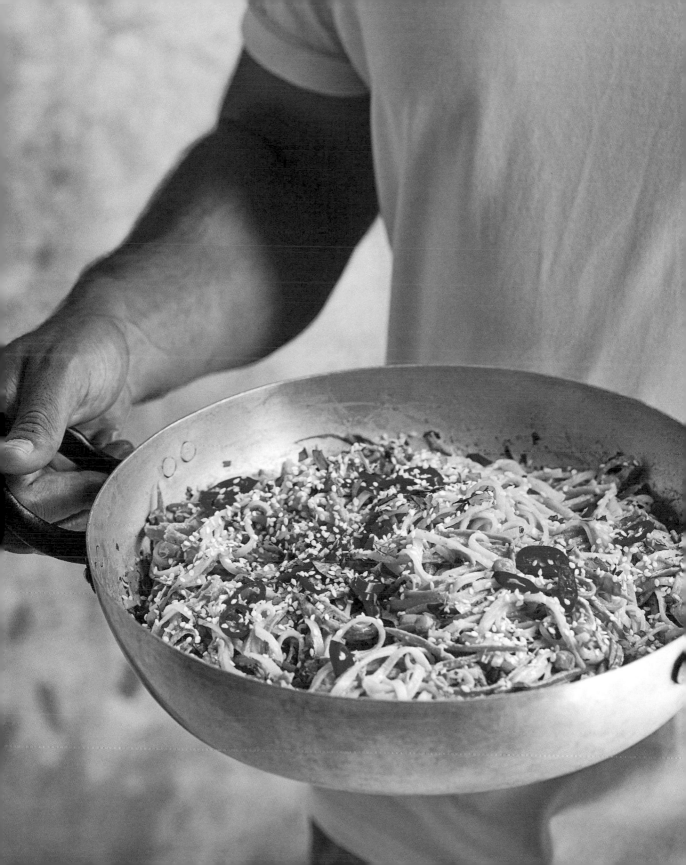

Sweet and sticky balsamic vinegar is one of my favourite flavours. I love using it with pine nuts and rosemary: the combination is simple yet effective.

Balsamic Sautéed Mushrooms with Rosemary

1 Heat a large frying pan over a medium to high heat. Drizzle the slices of bread with oil and fry for a minute or two on each side until golden. Remove from the pan and set aside.

2 Add 2 tablespoons of oil to the pan and sauté the mushrooms for 5 minutes.

3 Add the garlic and pine nuts to the pan and fry for 2 minutes to colour, then add the vinegar, capers, rosemary and plenty of salt and pepper. Cook for a further minute.

4 Finally, stir in the cavolo nero and cook for 2–3 minutes until tender.

5 Serve the sautéed mushrooms on the golden toast.

Cook's tip

Toast the bread instead of frying it, and serve it with a drizzle of olive oil.

PREP 5 MINUTES/COOK 10 MINUTES

2 thick slices of sourdough bread

3 tbsp extra-virgin olive oil, plus extra for drizzling

160g mix of shiitake mushrooms and oyster mushrooms, roughly ripped up

2 garlic cloves, thinly sliced

60g pine nuts

2 tbsp balsamic vinegar

30g capers, drained and rinsed

2–3 sprigs of rosemary

160g trimmed cavolo nero, shredded

sea salt and freshly ground black pepper

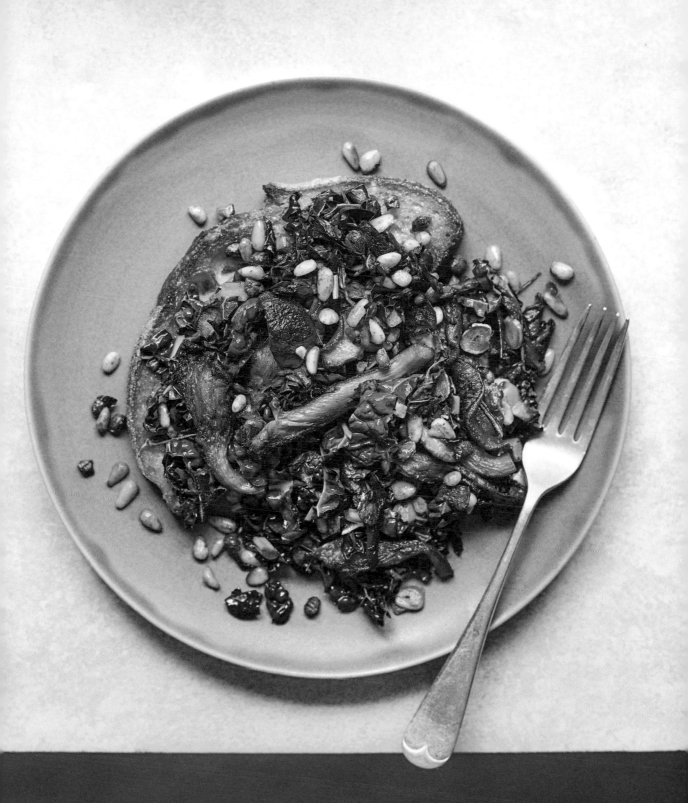

I love this twist on a takeaway favourite of mine. Instead of deep-frying the cauliflower in batter, you can get a beautiful flavour using a blend of sweet sauces (as well as sriracha, which packs quite a punch).

Bang Bang Cauliflower

1 Remove the leaves from the cauliflower and chop them roughly, then break the cauliflower into 2–3cm florets.

2 Mix the sauces, ginger, lime zest, juice and 100ml water together in a bowl.

3 Heat the sesame oil in a large wok or frying pan over a medium heat, add the onion and cauliflower leaves and fry for 5 minutes until golden.

4 Add the cauliflower florets and stir-fry for 3 minutes until coloured.

5 Add the sauce mix and cook for a further 5–6 minutes until the florets are tender.

6 Remove from the heat, stir through the beansprouts and serve scattered with coriander, peanuts and red chilli.

Variation

You could add some cooked tempeh or tofu with the cauliflower florets to make it a higher protein meal.

PREP 10 MINUTES/COOK 15 MINUTES

350g cauliflower (about ½ head or 1 small)
3 tbsp hoisin sauce
1 tbsp sriracha sauce
1 tbsp soy sauce
about 50g piece of root ginger (about 5cm), grated
finely grated zest and juice of 1 lime
1 tbsp sesame oil
160g red onion (about 1 medium), thinly sliced
100g beansprouts

TO SERVE
20g fresh coriander, finely chopped
60g unsalted peanuts, roughly chopped
1 red chilli, thinly sliced

The gorgeous flavours of fennel, coriander and lemon unite to deliver an amazing aromatic tone and earthiness to this simple sauté dish.

Green Beans and Black-eyed Peas

1 Heat the oil in a lidded sauté pan over a medium heat, add the onion and fry for 5 minutes until softened.

2 Add the green beans and spices, season with salt and pepper and cook for a further 2–3 minutes.

3 Toss in the spring greens and 2 tablespoons of water, cover and cook for 2–3 minutes until the greens are wilted and tender.

4 Stir through the black-eyed peas, cooking for 2 minutes to warm through, then fold in the parsley, add a squeeze of lemon juice and serve.

PREP 5 MINUTES/COOK 15 MINUTES

1 tbsp extra-virgin olive oil
100g red onion (about 1 small), thinly sliced
160g green beans
1 tsp fennel seeds
1 tsp coriander seeds, roughly crushed
1 tsp smoked sweet paprika
160g spring greens, thinly sliced
400g tin black-eyed peas, drained and rinsed
15g fresh flat-leaf parsley, chopped
squeeze of lemon juice
sea salt and freshly ground black pepper

Cook's tip

I sometimes use a touch of dried chilli flakes to add more heat.

Variation

Try using haricot beans, butter beans or cannellini in this recipe, instead of the black-eyed peas.

Miso, butter and mushrooms are a heavenly combination, and this dish is a super quick and easy way to put it to use.

Spring Vegetables with Miso Butter and Teriyaki Rice

1 Melt the miso paste and butter in a lidded wok or frying pan over a medium heat for a minute and whisk together. Add the chilli flakes, mushrooms and sesame seeds and stir-fry for 3–4 minutes.

2 Add the mangetout and asparagus to the wok with 1 tablespoon water. Cover and steam for 1–2 minutes, then uncover.

3 Add the teriyaki sauce and soy sauce and stir-fry for 2–3 minutes. Add the cooked rice and cook for 1–2 minutes more to heat through.

4 Remove from the heat and serve, scattered with the spring onions and the rest of the sesame seeds.

Cook's tip

You could easily add fish or chicken to this dish.

PREP 10 MINUTES/COOK 10 MINUTES

1 tbsp white miso paste
2 tbsp butter
1 tsp dried chilli flakes
100g shiitake mushrooms, torn
60g sesame seeds (reserve some for garnish)
160g mangetout
160g asparagus spears, roughly chopped
1 tbsp teriyaki sauce
1 tsp soy sauce
100g cooked brown rice
30g spring onions (about 2 or 3), thinly sliced

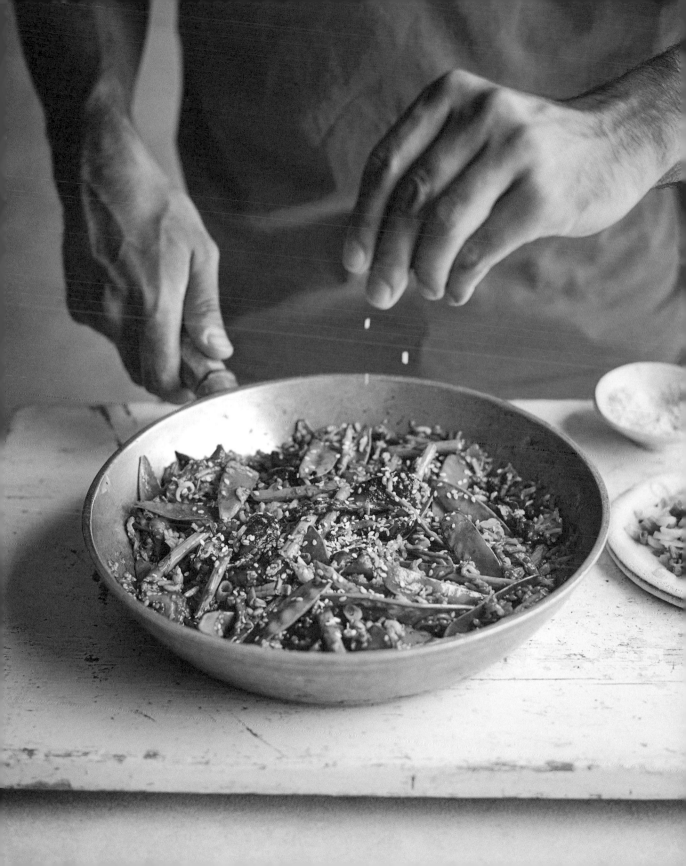

This takes me back to eating shawarmas late at night as a student. It's amazing how much flavour you can get out of some simple mushrooms when you use the right spices and pairings.

Spicy Mushroom and Tofu Shawarmas with Cucumber Yoghurt

1 Heat a wok or frying pan over a medium to high heat. Add the oil, mushrooms and tofu and fry for 7–8 minutes until browned all over.

2 Add the spices and pomegranate molasses, toss and cook for 2–3 minutes. Remove from the heat, toss in the cabbage and set aside.

3 For the cucumber yoghurt, mix the ingredients in a bowl and season.

4 Warm the flatbreads or pittas. Fill with the mushroom and cabbage mix and lots of cucumber and mint yoghurt. Add pickled peppers and hot sauce (if using).

Cook's tip

For an authentic cucumber yoghurt, salt the cucumber in a colander over a bowl. Toss and set aside for 15 minutes. Squeeze out the liquid, then add to the yoghurt.

Variation

Tempeh makes a more substantial alternative to firm tofu.

PREP 15 MINUTES/COOK 15 MINUTES

2 tbsp extra-virgin olive oil
160g mixed exotic mushrooms (oyster, king, shiitake), roughly torn
100g firm tofu, broken into 1.5cm chunks
1 tsp cumin seeds
½ tsp ground cinnamon
½ tsp ground coriander
½ tsp smoked sweet paprika
pinch of dried chilli flakes
1 tbsp pomegranate molasses
160g red cabbage (about ¼), very thinly sliced
Turkish flatbreads or pittas, to serve
30g pickled peppers (optional)
3 tsp hot sauce (optional)

FOR THE CUCUMBER YOGHURT
160g cucumber (about ½), coarsely grated
150g natural yoghurt (or soy-based)
1 garlic clove, grated
finely grated zest and juice of 1 lemon
20g fresh mint leaves, torn
sea salt and freshly ground black pepper

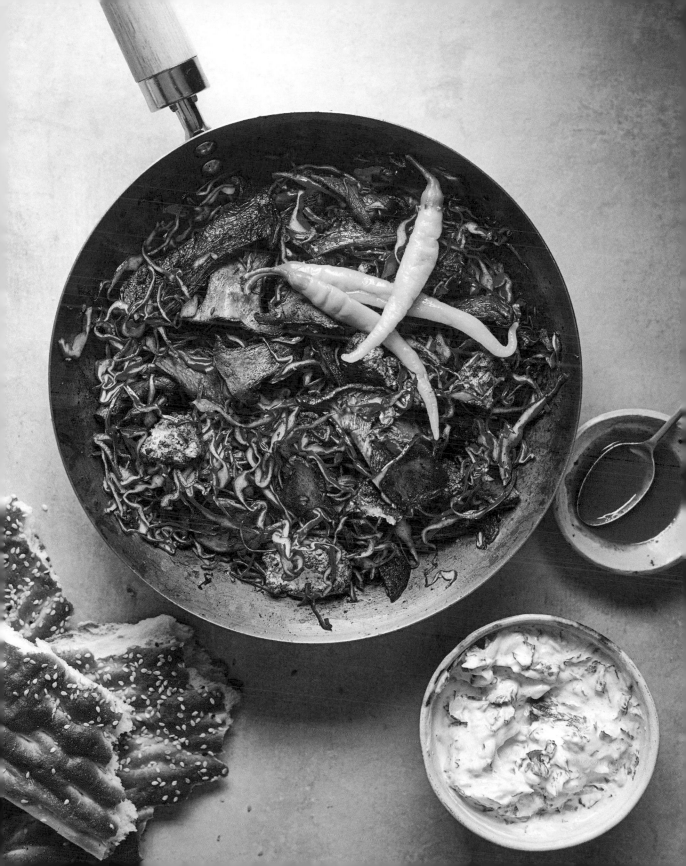

I use this quick tamari, soy and ginger mix for so many variations on this dish. It's punchy and super versatile.

Asian-style Green Vegetables in Black Bean Sauce

1 Whisk the garlic, ginger, tamari or soy sauce, and black bean paste in a bowl.

2 Heat the oil in a wok or frying pan over a medium heat. Add the peas and pak choi with the lemongrass and stir-fry for 5 minutes.

3 Add the garlic and ginger mixture, along with the black beans, and cook for a further 2–3 minutes.

4 Meanwhile, soak the noodles in boiling water for 10 minutes until tender, then drain and divide between two bowls.

5 Toss the water chestnuts through the stir-fry for a minute, then remove from the heat.

6 Spoon the stir-fry onto the noodles and scatter with the coriander and peanuts and a squeeze of lime juice.

PRE 10 MINUTES/COOK 10 MINUTES

2 garlic cloves, grated
25g piece of root ginger (about 2.5cm), grated
2 tbsp tamari or soy sauce
1 tbsp spicy black bean paste
1 tbsp sesame oil
160g sugar snap peas
160g pak choi, quartered
1 stick of lemongrass, bashed
400g tin black beans, drained and rinsed
100g vermicelli rice noodles
200g tin water chestnuts, drained, rinsed and chopped

TO SERVE
15g fresh coriander leaves, torn
20g unsalted peanuts, chopped
lime juice, to taste

Cook's tip

You can use a different chilli paste. Water chestnuts can also be replaced with regular cooked chestnuts.

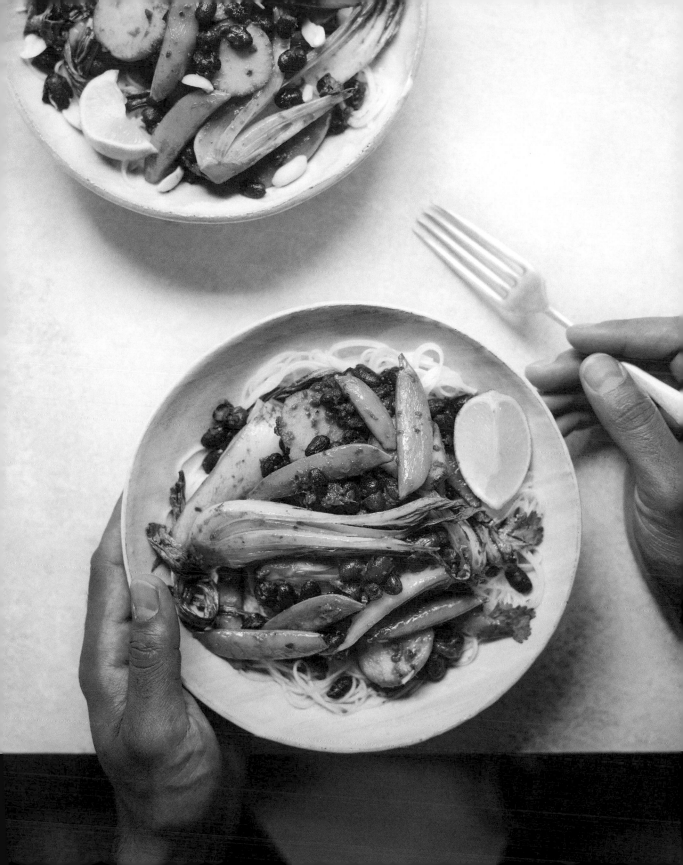

Index

References

Mills KT, Bundy JD, Kelly TN, et al. Global disparities of hypertension prevalence and control. Circulation. 2016. doi:10.1161/CIRCULATIONAHA.115.018912

Kurzer MS, Xu X. Dietary phytoestrogens. Annu Rev Nutr. 1997. doi:doi:10.1146/annurev.nutr.17.1.353

Peterson J, Dwyer J, Adlercreutz H, Scalbert A, Jacques P, McCullough ML. Dietary lignans: Physiology and potential for cardiovascular disease risk reduction. Nutr Rev. 2010. doi:10.1111/j.1753-4887.2010.00319.x

Williams C. Education and Debate Healthy Eating: Clarifying Advice about Fruit and Vegetables. Vol 310.; 1995.

Khaw KT, Wareham N, Bingham S, Welch A, Luben R, Day N. Combined impact of health behaviours and mortality in men and women: The EPIC-Norfolk prospective population study. PLoS Med. 2008;5(1):0039-0047. doi:10.1371/journal.pmed.0050012

Aune D, Giovannucci E, Boffetta P, et al. Fruit and vegetable intake and the risk of cardiovascular disease, total cancer and all-cause mortality – A systematic review and dose-response meta-analysis of prospective studies. Int J Epidemiol. 2017. doi:10.1093/ije/dyw319

Duthie SJ, Duthie GG, Russell WR, et al. Effect of increasing fruit and vegetable intake by dietary intervention on nutritional biomarkers and attitudes to dietary change: a randomised trial. Eur J Nutr. 2018. doi:10.1007/s00394-017-1469-0

Ludwig DS, Ebbeling CB, Heymsfield SB. Improving the Quality of Dietary Research. JAMA - J Am Med Assoc. 2019. doi:10.1001/jama.2019.11169

Malinowski B, Zalewska K, Węsierska A, et al. Intermittent fasting in cardiovascular disorders—an overview. Nutrients. 2019. doi:10.3390/nu11030673

Traba J, Geiger SS, Kwarteng-Siaw M, et al. Prolonged fasting suppresses mitochondrial NLRP3 inflammasome assembly and activation via SIRT3-mediated activation of superoxide dismutase 2. J Biol Chem. 2017. doi:10.1074/jbc.M117.791715

De Cabo R, Mattson MP. Effects of intermittent fasting on health, aging, and disease. N Engl J Med. 2019. doi:10.1056/NEJMra1905136

Lavin DN, Joesting JJ, Chiu GS, et al. Fasting induces an anti-inflammatory effect on the neuroimmune system which a high-fat diet prevents. Obesity. 2011. doi:10.1038/oby.2011.73

Yuan HX, Xiong Y, Guan KL. Nutrient Sensing, Metabolism, and Cell Growth Control. Mol Cell. 2013. doi:10.1016/j.molcel.2013.01.019

Lee JM, Wagner M, Xiao Y, et al. Nutrient-sensing nuclear receptors coordinate autophagy. Nature. 2014. doi:10.1038/nature13961

Maslowski KM, Vieira AT, Ng A, et al. Regulation of inflammatory responses by gut microbiota and chemoattractant receptor GPR43. Nature. 2009. doi:10.1038/nature08530

Vinolo MAR, Rodrigues HG, Nachbar RT, Curi R. Regulation of inflammation by short-chain fatty acids. Nutrients. 2011. doi:10.3390/nu3100858

Canani RB, Costanzo M Di, Leone L, Pedata M, Meli R, Calignano A. Potential beneficial effects of butyrate in intestinal and extraintestinal diseases. World J Gastroenterol. 2011. doi:10.3748/wjg.v17.i12.1519

Marlow G, Ellett S, Ferguson IR, et al. Transcriptomics to study the effect of a Mediterranean-inspired diet on inflammation in Crohn's disease patients. Hum Genomics. 2013. doi:10.1186/1479-7364-7-24

O'Keefe SJD, Li J V., Lahti L, et al. Fat, fibre and cancer risk in African Americans and rural Africans. Nat Commun. 2015. doi:10.1038/ncomms7342

Zinöcker MK, Lindseth IA. The western diet–microbiome-host interaction and its role in metabolic disease. Nutrients. 2018. doi:10.3390/nu10030365

Cordain L, Eaton SB, Sebastian A, et al. Origins and evolution of the Western diet: Health implications for the 21st century. Am J Clin Nutr. 2005.

Hodges RE, Minich DM. Modulation of Metabolic Detoxification Pathways Using Foods and Food-Derived Components: A Scientific Review with Clinical Application. J Nutr Metab. 2015. doi:10.1155/2015/760689

Jovanovski E, Bosco L, Khan K, et al. Effect of Spinach, a High Dietary Nitrate Source, on Arterial Stiffness and Related Hemodynamic Measures: A Randomized, Controlled Trial in Healthy Adults. Clin Nutr Res. 2015. doi:10.7762/cnr.2015.4.3.160

De Souza RGM, Schincaglia RM, Pimente GD, Mota JF. Nuts and human health outcomes: A systematic review. Nutrients. 2017. doi:10.3390/nu9121311

Ros E. Health benefits of nut consumption. Nutrients. 2010. doi:10.3390/nu2070652

Bao Y, Han J, Hu FB, et al. Association of nut consumption with total and cause-specific mortality. N Engl J Med. 2013. doi:10.1056/NEJMoa1307352

Bohlooli S, Barmaki S, Khoshkhahesh F, Nakhostin-Roohi B. The effect of spinach supplementation on exercise-induced oxidative stress. J Sports Med Phys Fitness. 2015.

Zhang JJ, Li Y, Zhou T, et al. Bioactivities and health benefits of mushrooms mainly from China. Molecules. 2016. doi:10.3390/molecules21070938

Roberts JL, Moreau R. Functional properties of spinach (Spinacia oleracea L.) phytochemicals and bioactives. Food Funct. 2016. doi:10.1039/c6fo00051g

Kristal AR, Lampe JW. Brassica vegetables and prostate cancer risk: A review of the epidemiological evidence. Nutr Cancer. 2002. doi:10.1207/S15327914NC421_1

Verhoeven DTH, Goldbohm RA, Van Poppel G, Verhagen H, Van Den Brandt PA. Epidemiological studies on Brassica vegetables and cancer risk. Cancer Epidemiol Biomarkers Prev. 1996.

González-Peña D, Checa A, de Ancos B, Wheelock CE, Sánchez-Moreno C. New insights into the effects of onion consumption on lipid mediators using a diet-induced model of hypercholesterolemia. Redox Biol. 2017. doi:10.1016/j.redox.2016.12.002

Butt MS, Sultan MT, Butt MS, Iqbal J. Garlic: Nature's protection against physiological threats. Crit Rev Food Sci Nutr. 2009. doi:10.1080/10408390802145344

Griffiths G, Trueman L, Crowther T, Thomas B, Smith B. Onions - A global benefit to health. Phyther Res. 2002. doi:10.1002/ptr.1222

Carlson JL, Erickson JM, Lloyd BB, Slavin JL. Health effects and sources of prebiotic dietary fiber. Curr Dev Nutr. 2018. doi:10.1093/cdn/nzy005

Ahmadi S, Mainali R, Nagpal R, et al. Dietary Polysaccharides in the Amelioration of Gut Microbiome Dysbiosis and Metabolic Diseases. Obes Control Ther. open access. 2017.

Bruznican S, De Clercq H, Eeckhaut T, Van Huylenbroeck J, Geelen D. Celery and Celeriac: A Critical View on Present and Future Breeding. Front Plant Sci. 2020. doi:10.3389/fpls.2019.01699

Acknowledgements

To my mum, dad and sister whose love and support allow me to chase my ambitions. I know you would prefer I take the easy route, but life's not fun without adventure, wonder and dreams. To my girlfriend who has to put up with so much. Thank you allowing me the time and headspace to be creative and whacky (… and annoying) in the pursuit of something much bigger than me. And thank you for bringing Nutmeg into our lives. She really is the cutest 'pupperoo, that never grew'.

To my closest friends and my online community whose messages and gestures of support over the last 5 years have kept me pushing The Doctor's Kitchen inch by inch. Your backing and belief in the mission is what keeps me driving forward and I cannot thank you all enough. This is all because of your love.

To my wonderful publishing team at Thorsons/HarperCollins UK, the photography, food writing and styling crew and my amazing literary agent, Carly Cook, for their incredible support. Thank you so much for your continual belief in the mission and for trusting me so much with this concept. And to Stuart Renshaw and the team at Whisk, thank you for making this book even more accessible with your digital extension. It's very much appreciated.

To my Culinary Medicine UK team who continue to bear the torch for a project that will change the way nutrition is developed, taught and practiced by all medical practitioners. Thank you for tirelessly supporting the mission. I promise it will be worth it.

To the scientists in the field of nutritional research whose work forms the very backbone of The Doctor's Kitchen and the reason as to why I can confidently prescribe and talk about food and lifestyle as medicine. You are the unsung heroes of a movement that should have started decades ago. A special shout to all health professionals transforming the way they practice and becoming beacons of a movement that embraces food and lifestyle as medicine. Together we will revolutionise wellbeing and healthcare for the better and overcome the critics who merely spectate from the side lines. We can do this.

To my patients who teach me as much as I am able to help them. I'm fortunate to still practice in our national healthcare system and to care for people in their most vulnerable state. For this most privileged of positions, I am so grateful.

I also want to thank myself. I know that sounds incredibly narcissistic, but I'm the type of person who suffers classic imposter syndrome and I'm plagued with self-doubt. I rarely indulge in the opportunity to thank myself and reflect on the hard work it takes to build and nurture an online community, write books, release podcasts, start a non-profit organisation, create recipes, teach medical students, develop digital platforms and practice medicine. You're doing a good thing Rupy. Keep it up.